HEALTH EMERGENCY PLANNING:

A Handbook for Practitioners

EDITED BY
Sarah Norman, Jim Stuart-Black and Eve Coles

FOREWORD BY
;el Lightfoot

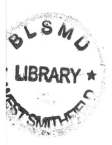

TSO: London

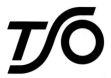

Published by TSO (The Stationery Office) and available from:

Online
www.tsoshop.co.uk

Mail, Telephone, Fax & E-mail
TSO
PO Box 29, Norwich, NR3 1GN
Telephone orders/General enquiries: 0870 600 5522
Fax orders: 0870 600 5533
E-mail: customer.services@tso.co.uk
Textphone 0870 240 3701

TSO Shops
123 Kingsway, London, WC2B 6PQ
020 7242 6393 Fax 020 7242 6394
68-69 Bull Street, Birmingham B4 6AD
0121 236 9696 Fax 0121 236 9699
9-21 Princess Street, Manchester M60 8AS
0161 834 7201 Fax 0161 833 0634
16 Arthur Street, Belfast BT1 4GD
028 9023 8451 Fax 028 9023 5401
18-19 High Street, Cardiff CF10 1PT
029 2039 5548 Fax 029 2038 4347
71 Lothian Road, Edinburgh EH3 9AZ
0870 606 5566 Fax 0870 606 5588

TSO Accredited Agents
(see Yellow Pages)

and through good booksellers

First published 2006

ISBN 0 11 703246 8
13 digit ISBN 978 0 11 703246 0

Printed in the United Kingdom for The Stationery Office
N186685 C10 04/06 334264 19585

Contents

Figures

Tables

Boxes

Acronyms

A

A&E   Accident and Emergency (Department)
ACCOLC   Access Overload Control (for cellular radio telephones)
ACPO   Association of Chief Police Officers
ACPO TAM   The Terrorism and Allied Matters Committee of ACPO
AIO   Ambulance Incident Officer
ASA   Ambulance Service Association
ASO   Ambulance Safety Officer
ATC   Air traffic control
AWE   Atomic Weapons Establishment

B

BLT   St Bartholomew's and the Royal London Trust
Bq   Becquerel
BT   British Telecom
BTS   Blood Transfusion Service

C

CAA   Civil Aviation Authority
CACFOA   Chief and Assistant Chief Fire Officers Association
CAM   Chemical agent monitor
CAMR   Centre for Applied Medical Research
CAOC   Combined Air Operations Centre
CBIED   Chemical, biological improvised explosive device
CBRN   Chemical, biological, radiological and nuclear
CCC   Civil Contingencies Committee
CCDC   Consultant in communicable disease control
CCS   Civil Contingencies Secretariat
CDC   Communicable disease control
CDR   Classified document register
CDSC   Communicable Disease Surveillance Centre
CHAPs   Chemical Hazards and Poisons (Division of the Health Protection Agency)
CIMAH   Control of Industrial Major Accident Hazards Regulations 1984
CMO   Chief Medical Officer
CNI   Critical national infrastructure
COBR   Cabinet Office Briefing Room
COMAH   Control of Major Accident Hazards Regulations 1999
CRR   Community risk register

D

Defra   Department for Environment, Food and Rural Affairs
DH   Department of Health
DPH   Director of Public Health (in a Primary Care Trust)
DSTL   Defence Scientific Testing Laboratory

DTI	Department of Trade and Industry
DTLR	Department for Transport, Local Government and the Regions

E

EBS	Emergency Bed Service
ECHR	European Convention on Human Rights
ECN	Emergency communication network
EHO	Environmental Health Officer
EMA	Emergency Management Australia
EOD	Explosive ordinance disposal
EPCU	The Department of Health's Emergency Planning Coordination Unit (now renamed the Health Emergency Preparedness Division)
EPD	Emergency Preparedness Division (a division of the Department of Health)
EPLO	Emergency Planning Liaison Officer
ERA	Elected Regional Assembly

F

FAA	Federal Aviation Administration
FCO	Foreign & Commonwealth Office

G

GLO	Government Liaison Officer
GLT	Government Liaison Team
GMS	Global messaging system (phones)
GNN	Government News Network
GO	Government office
GORs	Government Office Regions
GTA	Government Technical Adviser
GTPS	Government telephone preference scheme
Gy	Gray

H

HAGCCI	Health Advisory Group on Chemical Contamination Incidents
HAT	Health Advice Team
HAZMAT	Hazardous materials
HEPA	Health Emergency Planning Adviser (regional)
HMCIFS	HM Chief Inspector of Fire Services
HSE	Health and Safety Executive

I

IEM	Integrated emergency management
ILO	Inter-agency Liaison Officer (Fire Service)
IPE	Individual protective equipment (military)
IPPC	Integrated Pollution Prevention and Control
ITU	Intensive treatment unit

J

JESCC	Joint Emergency Services Control Centre
JHAC	Joint Health Advisory Cell

L

LAEPO	Local Authority Emergency Planning Officer
LaRS	Local and Regional Services (Division of the Health Protection Agency)
LAS	London Ambulance Service
LEC	Local emergency centre
LESLP	London Emergency Services Liaison Panel
LFEPA	London Fire Emergency Planning Authority
LGA	Local Government Association
LRF	Local Resilience Forum

M

MACA	Military assistance to the civil authority
MACC	Military aid to the civil community
MACP	Military aid to the civil power
MAFF	Ministry of Agriculture, Fisheries and Food (now Defra)
MAGD	Military aid to other government departments
MCA	Military or Ministry of Defence Coordinating Authority
MEC	Medical evacuation cell (military)
MIO	Medical Incident Officer
MMT	Mobile Medical Team
MOD	Ministry of Defence
mSv	Millisievert (one thousandth of a sievert)
µSv	Microsievert (one millionth of a sievert)

N

NAIR	National arrangements for incidents involving radioactivity
NAO	National Audit Office
NBC	Nuclear, biological and chemical
NCC	News Co-ordination Centre
NEBR	Nuclear Emergency Briefing Room
NFCI	National focus for chemical incidents
NHS	National Health Service
NPIS	National Poisons Information Service
NRPB	National Radiological Protection Board

O

ODPM	Office of the Deputy Prime Minister
OECD	Organisation for Economic Cooperation and Development

P

PCT	Primary Care Trust
PGDs	Patient Group Directives
PHLS	Public Health Laboratory Service
POLSA	Police Search Adviser
POST	Parliamentary Office of Science and Technology
PPE	Personal protective equipment

R

RAMP	Reception arrangements for military patients
RAYNET	Radio Amateurs Emergency Network
RCCC	Regional Civil Contingencies Committee
RDsPH	Regional Directors of Public Health
RHEPA	Regional Health Emergency Planning Adviser
RIMNET	Radioactive Incident Monitoring Network
RMEF	Regional Media Emergency Forum
RPD	Radiological Protection Division (of the Health Protection Agency)
RSPU	Regional service provider unit (for advice on chemical incident response)
RTA	Road traffic accident

S

SCG	Strategic Coordinating Group
SEPA	Scottish Environmental Protection Agency
SHA	Strategic Health Authority
SMS	Short Message (or Messaging) Service/System in Global Messaging Service/System (GMS)(cellular phones)
SRMD	Specialist and Reference Microbiology Division
STEP 123	Safety Triggers for Emergency Personnel
Sv	Sievert

T

TPU	Terrorism and Protection Unit (Home Office)

U

UKSRR	United Kingdom Search and Rescue Region (of the Maritime and Coastguard Agency)
UN	United Nations
USAR	Urban search and rescue (fire)

V

VAS	Voluntary aid societies

W

WHO	World Health Organisation

Notes on contributors

Eve Coles

Eve Coles is Senior Lecturer in Risk and Emergency Management in the Coventry University Centre for Disaster Management. She began her academic life as administrator/researcher for the Disaster Prevention and Limitation Unit (DPLU), based at the University of Bradford, where she helped organise and run the annual DPLU international conferences on disaster management and emergency planning. From Bradford she worked for seven years with Professor Denis Smith, in his Centre for Risk and Crisis Management, before joining Coventry University. She is a Fellow of the Institute of Civil Defence and Disaster Studies, and a member of the European Sociological Society and the International Research Committee on Disasters. She was formally editor of *Emergency*, the quarterly journal of the Institute of Civil Defence & Disaster Studies. Her research interests include emergency management policy and emergency planning in local authorities in the UK, with particular interest in professional qualifications and the core skills and competencies of local authority emergency planners; business continuity management for public sector organisations; and the use of the internet as an information and communication resource in the management of emergencies and disasters. In her spare time Eve is vice-chair of governors at a Bradford primary school, a post she has held for 13 years.

Ann Fleming

Ann Fleming has managed crisis communications in the public sector with sustained international and national media attention. She currently works in the West Midlands for the Health Protection Agency.

Nigel Lightfoot

Dr Nigel Lightfoot is the Director of Emergency Response, located at the Health Protection Agency (HPA) Centre for Emergency Preparedness and Response at Porton Down, Wiltshire. Dr Lightfoot is responsible for emergency preparedness within the HPA for CBRN threats and for coordinating the assets of the HPA during such emergencies. In addition to his principal role, Dr Lightfoot is also Director, HPA Influenza and Respiratory Viruses Programme Board, Co-Chair of the Risk Management and Co-ordination Working Group of the Global Health Security Action Group of the G7, and he is an adviser to the Ministry of Defence on medical countermeasures and CBRN matters.

Originally qualifying at St Mary's Medical School, University College, London, in 1968, Dr Lightfoot served with the Royal Navy for 13 years, going on to gain an MSc Med Micro (1976) and his MRCPath (1979), before moving to become a Consultant Adviser in Medical Microbiology. Spending some 20 years in the Public Health Service as a consultant medical microbiologist, Dr Lightfoot has published over 100 papers covering a range of topics including bioterrorism, dangerous pathogens, anthrax and tularaemia, and a number of public health issues. Seconded to the Department of Health in 2002, Dr Lightfoot joined the HPA on its inception in 2003.

Jill Meara

Dr Meara went to medical school in Cambridge and Oxford. After general professional training she specialised in public health, working in Oxford and gaining an MSc from the London School of Hygiene and Tropical Medicine. She spent 10 years as Director of Public Health for Northamptonshire, where she dealt with a number of 'environmental' incidents and concerns, including a cluster of childhood leukaemia near a railway line and depleted uranium fly-tipped on farmland. In 2000 she joined the National Radiological Protection Board (now the Radiological Protection Division of HPA) as its first ever Public Health Physician. At the Radiological Protection Division she has a remit to improve the way the division works with statutory agencies and the public. She is a fellow of the Faculty of Public Health.

Dilys Morgan

Dr Morgan is Consultant Epidemiologist at the Communicable Disease Surveillance Centre (CDSC) of the Health Protection Agency, and is currently responsible for bioterrorism response and emerging infections. She was in charge of the investigation and management of outbreaks of communicable diseases at CDSC from 1992 to 1995, before going to work in Africa. She spent the next six years working for the Medical Research Council as a clinical epidemiologist, researching the natural history of HIV infection in rural Uganda, before returning to work in the HIV division of CDSC in May 2001.

Les Moseley

Les is Director of the Coventry University Centre for Disaster Management. He is also Head of the Disaster Management subject group and Programme Manager for all professional development courses. Before joining Coventry University, Les spent 16 years in the British Fire Service, as a senior officer, and 14 years in emergency planning; he was also County Emergency Planning Officer for Warwickshire County Council, and Chief Emergency Planning Officer and Principal Officer with the West Midlands Fire and Civil Defence Authority. His current (funded) research is focused towards the use of training and validation techniques for strategic and tactical management of major emergencies and crisis management, and the use of current and future technology to improve the response to, and management of, major transport incidents. Les is an active member of the Emergency Planning Society and the Institute of Civil Defence and Disaster Studies, and is currently chairman of the south Midlands branch of the institute.

Virginia Murray

Dr Murray is Consultant Medical Toxicologist in the Chemical Hazards and Poisons (CHAPs) Division of the Health Protection Agency. She trained in occupational medicine before joining the National Poisons Information Service, London, and the Medical Toxicology Unit, in 1980. In 1989 she started the Chemical Incident Research Programme and has been Director of the Chemical Incident Response Service since 1996. This service supported, via service level agreements, all health protection units in six and a half of the nine regions. (On 1 April 2003 this service became part of the Health Protection Agency.) As a result, she has considerable experience in advising on the toxicological aspects of response to chemical incidents.

Sarah Norman

Originally from New Zealand, Sarah trained as a Registered Comprehensive Nurse before moving to the UK and undertaking extensive travel in Europe, the Middle East and Africa. In 2000 she completed a BSc (Hons) in Development and Health in Disaster Management, before travelling to Ethiopia to work as the Monitoring and Evaluation Officer for Concern Worldwide during the 2000 food crisis. Following a return to Coventry University in 2001 to complete an MSc (by research) in Disaster Management, she became a Regional Health Emergency Planning Adviser in London. Sarah is currently employed as an Emergency Management Planner by the Ministry of Civil Defence and Emergency Management in Wellington, New Zealand.

Jim Stuart-Black

After a number of years working overseas, Jim returned to the UK and completed a BA (Hons) degree in Disaster Management. Upon graduation, he took up the post of Emergency Planning and Security Manager for the London Borough of Havering, and was an active member of the Emergency Planning Society (London branch) and the Institute of Civil Defence & Disaster Studies, winning the 2002 Sir John Hodsall essay-writing competition. Jim is currently employed as the National Manager, Special Operations, with the New Zealand Fire Service. Jim regularly lectures on various emergency management programmes in New Zealand, and maintains an active research interest in the area of individual and collective decision making in emergency situations.

Foreword

For some time there has been a need for a textbook on health emergency planning. It is now here and will be required reading for all those involved in planning for or responding to health emergencies. From my perspective, the first half of this decade has revealed health emergency preparedness to be an extremely complex area, one that of necessity involves many diverse stakeholders, a number of whom are not health-care organisations. Experience has proven that, without exception, major incidents or associated emergencies will include an element of health involvement during the incident. It is also a fact that recent major incidents, resulting in physical injury to victims, have required health input from the onset of the incident, through secondary and tertiary care regimes, until the patient has either succumbed to their injuries or realised a successful outcome. In other words, from the arrival of the Ambulance Service at the incident, the injured victim enters the health-care continuum and will remain within that continuum until treatment has been completed. This can last for a considerable time and does not only apply to physically injured victims – those who are psychosocially affected will also require considerable assistance from the health-care fraternity, and must be followed up appropriately for some time.

However, concurrent with responding to the needs of the incident, health organisations have to ensure, in terms of emergency preparedness, that they maintain health resilience and continue to provide a comprehensive health service to the general public. Members of the public will still suffer acute and chronic life-threatening conditions and illnesses that may require immediate and complicated treatment, despite the fact that a major incident is in progress in their near vicinity. These patients will require the services of paramedics and the staff in A&E and other departments of the Acute Trust that is receiving victims from the major incident.

I describe this essentially to reinforce the complexities of health emergency preparedness – complexities that I believe differ from those faced by our colleagues in the non-health organisations and agencies who also have a major role to play in emergency preparedness. For instance, in the capital and large metropolitan areas, the ambulance control could arrange for another nearby hospital to take non-incident patients for treatment, but in rural areas, where acute hospitals may be 30 to 40 miles apart, that option is not so easy and hospital capacity becomes a major planning concern. This is business continuity, you might say, and I would agree; however, it must go much further than the basic concepts of business continuity, because in health terms, if our day-to-day business is disrupted, we need to ensure that we not only maintain a service, but that we do so with a large number of uncertainties to factor into our planning, into our preparedness if you will.

Therefore, when we consider that, in parallel to planning for the recognised man-made or influenced incidents, which include terrorism, health planners also have to incorporate pandemics, epidemics, environmental incidents and incidents of a non-traumatic or life-threatening nature. When this affects the capability and capacity of a large Acute Trust or health-care facility, then the complexities involved in planning become far more intricate. We have all learned from recent events that multi-agency responses are essential, and that working on a multi-agency basis in the preparedness phase has immense value on the day. I welcome the introduction of the Civil

Contingencies Act and its accompanying regulations, which will do much to involve health further in the multi-agency emergency planning arena. This book will be an essential desktop companion to those involved in planning in the health emergency field.

The editors and contributors are to be congratulated on producing a most comprehensive and informative work. Thus, I welcome the publication of this handbook and commend it without reservation to all involved or associated with the discipline of health emergency planning.

Dr Nigel Lightfoot

Preface

Health Emergency Planning: A Handbook for Practitioners is designed as a resource tool which can be used by emergency planners in a health context to provide practical advice, ideas, resources and references to facilitate emergency planning. The handbook provides some of the fundamental concepts of emergency planning whilst also encouraging readers to strive for best practice. For more specific guidance on the roles and responsibilities of health-care providers, practitioners should refer to the Department of Health (2005) publication, *The NHS Emergency Planning Guidance.*

This publication has been prepared for the Health Protection Agency Centre for Emergency Preparedness and Response. It is aimed at all aspects of the health emergency planning profession, including Health Emergency Planning Officers and all those who commission health emergency planning: this will include the chief executives and those charged with the responsibility for emergency planning within Strategic Health Authorities, Primary Care Trusts, Acute Trusts, Ambulance Trusts, Specialist Trusts and Mental Health Trusts. Regional Health Emergency Planning Advisers may use the handbook as a resource and support document. It may also prove useful to emergency planners engaged in related fields, including local authorities, emergency services and those studying in complementary disciplines. The authors anticipate that this handbook will prove to be a well-thumbed reference for all health emergency practitioners keen to develop their skills and knowledge in a newly developing profession.

The handbook begins with an introduction to major incidents and disasters, and provides an overview, in Chapter 2, of the legal framework that drives the emergency planning process. Crisis management and organisational learning – including the culture of organisations – are then introduced in Chapter 3, which encourages the practitioner to promote emergency planning and preparedness as part of day-to-day work practice.

Hazard identification and risk management are explored in Chapter 4, which also provides both practical advice and a user-friendly model. The concept of emergency plans is explained in Chapter 5, including the types of plans, their structure and the planning process. To complete the plan process, Chapter 6 explores the auditing and reviewing of plans, and Chapter 7 addresses training and exercises.

The multi-agency response is clearly documented in Chapter 8, to encourage readers to understand fully the context within which they work, as the different agencies may be operating in support of a major incident declared by and affecting your own organisation alone, or, as will often be the case, you will be operating in support of other agencies as part of an overarching strategic framework. The health response is outlined separately in Chapter 9, which covers the roles and responsibilities of the Department of Health, the Health Protection Agency and the National Health Service, as well as the relationships that exist from local to national level within the health-care economy.

Building on these core concepts, Chapter 10 of the handbook reflects the current climate of terrorist threat by providing a chapter on chemical, biological, radiological and nuclear (CBRN) incidents. The reader is given practical advice on what should be in CBRN and mass casualty plans, and how to identify such events and recognise cases of unusual illness. Decontamination, sheltering and evacuation are also explored. For more specific guidance on CBRN incidents, practitioners should continue to refer to the Department of Health (2000) publication, *Deliberate Release of Biological and Chemical Agents: Guidance to Help Plan the Health Service's Response,* the Home Office (2004) publication, *The Decontamination of People Exposed to Chemical, Biological, Radiological or Nuclear (CBRN) Substances or Materials: Strategic National Guidance* and the HPA (2005) publication by Heptonstall and Gent, *CBRN Incidents: Clinical Management and Health Protection.*

Planning for public relations and media management is extensively explained in Chapter 11, with practical guidance on how to prepare a media plan, planning interviews and news conferences, and understanding the flow of information. The final chapter explains organisational debriefing and reporting following major incidents, and suggests possible support mechanisms that can be offered to staff. Finally, a full glossary and annexes of supporting documents are provided.

Important points for the reader to note:

- this is a handbook, rather than a textbook
- the handbook is a collection of related papers written by a number of authors
- the handbook is not intended to read as though one author had written it
- the handbook acts as a supporting resource to the Department of Health (2005) publication, *The NHS Emergency Planning Guidance*
- the handbook offers help and support to practitioners new to emergency planning by providing practical advice.

Acknowledgements

We would like to thank the following people for their invaluable contributions in the preparation and production of this handbook: Les Moseley (Coventry University Centre for Disaster Management); Virginia Murray (Chemical Hazards and Poisons [CHAPs] Division, Health Protection Agency); Dilys Morgan (Health Protection Agency); Jill Meara (Radiological Protection Division); Jonathan Asbridge (St Bartholomew's and the Royal London Hospital Trust); Mark Avery (Whittington Hospital Trust, London); Charles Blanch (London Fire and Emergency Planning Authority); Philip Buckle (Coventry University Centre for Disaster Management); Richard Cocks (Regional HEPA, Health Protection Agency); Steve Conway (Regional HEPA for Scotland); Adrian Cooper; Lawrence Davies (Regional HEPA, Health Protection Agency); Mathew Drinkwater (CHAPs Division, Health Protection Agency); Adrienne Edkins (CHAPs Division, Health Protection Agency); Ann Fleming (Health Protection Agency); David Goulding (Regional HEPA for Wales); Tracey Grant (Regional Health Emergency Planning Assistant, London); Chris Gundry (Regional HEPA, Health Protection Agency); John Handmer (RMIT, Melbourne, Australia); Andrew Healy (Regional HEPA, Health Protection Agency); Gareth Holt (Regional HEPA, Health Protection Agency); Peter Kendal (Regional HEPA, Health Protection Agency); Laurence Knight (Health Protection Agency Central Office); Dr Nigel Lightfoot (Emergency Response Division, Health Protection Agency); Mick Messenger (Metropolitan Police Service); Richard Middleton and Matthew Moran (TSO [The Stationery Office]); Liz Morgan-Lewis (Health Protection Agency); Raji Nandipati (CHAPs Division, Health Protection Agency); Dr Margo Nicols (CHAPs Division, Health Protection Agency); Tim Pettis (Strategic Emergency Planning Manager, Health Protection Agency); Dr John Simpson (Emergency Response Division, Health Protection Agency); Michele Staple (TSO); Phil Storr (Regional HEPA, Health Protection Agency); Peter Szekley (Department of Health); Dave Ward (Regional HEPA, Health Protection Agency); Sarah Webb (Regional HEPA, Health Protection Agency); Sue Wheatley (Regional HEPA, Health Protection Agency) and Amanda Welsh (CHAPs Division, Health Protection Agency). We would particularly like to thank Gordon MacDonald, Head of Strategic Emergency Planning, HPA, for his support during the completion of this project.

Sarah Norman, Jim Stuart-Black and Eve Coles

February 2006

1

Introduction to Major Incidents and Disasters

Eve Coles

1.1 Introduction

This chapter is essentially an informative one, which will attempt to clarify what a disaster/major incident is and how the concept of 'integrated emergency management' was adopted as a framework for dealing with such incidents in the UK. It includes sections on:

- definitions of disaster
- disasters to major incidents
- understanding disasters
- the disaster cycle
- integrated emergency planning.

Disasters can be very complex events, as indeed is the definitional debate that surrounds them. Similarly, the way disasters are described and dealt with in the UK is also complex, as the Cabinet Office (2003) points out: 'No single organisational arrangement will be appropriate to each and every disaster, nor will a single organisational planning blueprint meet every need. The key to an effective response is to apply sound principles, founded on experience, to the problem in hand.' Part of that effective response is a clear understanding of disaster and all it implies.

1.2 Definitions

1.2.1 Major incidents

A disaster is commonly understood to be a great misfortune or calamity, and a negative event. In the context of civil protection a useful working definition of a disaster is:

> ... any event (happening with or without warning) causing or threatening death or injury, damage to property or to the environment or disruption to the community, which because of the scale of its effects cannot be dealt with by the emergency services and local authorities as part of their day-to-day activities (Cabinet Office 2003).

Within the emergency services the term 'major incident' is used rather than disaster, since there are specific events that will initiate a response under the framework of the services' major incident plan. The following definition is set out in the Association of Chief Police Officers' Emergency Procedures Manual and in the Fire Service's Major Incident Emergency Procedures Manual:

> A major incident is any emergency that requires the implementation of special arrangements by one or more of the emergency services, the NHS or the local authority for:
>
> - the initial treatment, rescue and transport of a large number of casualties

- the involvement either directly or indirectly of large numbers of people
- the handling of a large number of enquiries likely to be generated both from the public and the news media, usually to the police
- the need for the large-scale combined resources of two or more of the emergency services
- the mobilisation and organisation of the emergency services and supporting organisations, e.g. local authority, to cater for the threat of death, serious injury or homelessness to a large number of people (Cabinet Office 2003).

The broad definition above is also applicable to the NHS, as the wording indicates. For specific NHS purposes, a major incident may be defined as:

> Any occurrence which presents a serious threat to the health of the community, disruption to the service, or causes (or is likely to cause) such numbers or types of casualties as to require special arrangements to be implemented by hospitals, ambulance services or health authorities (Cabinet Office 2003).

The Department of Health (2004) document, *Handling Major Incidents: An Operational Doctrine*, builds on the above definition of a major incident, stating:

> Each individual NHS organisation must plan to handle incidents in which its own facilities – or neighbouring ones – may be overwhelmed. Planning successfully for these wider disruptive challenges will require more than simply scaling up the current plans of individual agencies.

The document also acknowledges the need for the scale of major incidents to be considered, as follows:

- Trusts in the NHS are accustomed to normal fluctuations in daily demand for services (peaks and troughs). Whilst at times this may lead to facilities being fully stretched, such fluctuations are managed without the activation of special measures.

- Individual Ambulance Services or Trusts are also well-versed in handling incidents such as multi-vehicle motorway crashes within long-established 'major accident plans'.

Beyond this, two levels can usefully be described:

- Level II incidents – much larger scale events affecting potentially hundreds rather than tens of people, possibly also involving the closure or evacuation of a major facility (e.g. because of fire or contamination) or persistent disruption over many days; these will require a collective response by several or many neighbouring Trusts.

- Level III incidents – events of potentially catastrophic proportions that severely disrupt health and social care and other functions (power, water, etc.) and that exceed even collective capability within the NHS (Department of Health 2004).

The National Audit Office (NAO) (2003) publication, *Facing the Challenge: NHS Emergency Planning in England*, defines a major incident as:

> ... any emergency that requires the implementation of special arrangements by one or more of the emergency services, the NHS, or the local authority. For the NHS, a major incident is any occurrence which

presents a serious threat to the health of the community, disruption to the service, or causes (or is likely to cause) such numbers or types of casualties as to require special arrangements to be implemented by hospitals, ambulance services or Primary Care Trusts.

Major incidents may take many forms, for example:

- Chemical:
  - technological, e.g. the chemical disaster in Bhopal, India
  - deliberate, e.g. the sarin attack in Tokyo
  - accidental, e.g. a motor vehicle accident involving a tanker carrying chemicals.
- Biological:
  - new or re-emerging organisms, e.g. SARS or HIV
  - epi- or pandemics, e.g. influenza or SARS
  - failure of routine therapy and/or development of antibiotic resistance, e.g. MRSA
  - failure of vaccination programme, e.g. measles, mumps and rubella (MMR), pertussis
  - deliberate, e.g. smallpox or plague.
- Radiological/nuclear:
  - accident, e.g. Chernobyl
  - natural, e.g. radon
  - deliberate, e.g. dirty bomb.
- Natural/environmental:
  - earthquakes
  - weather, e.g. flooding
  - volcanoes
  - subsidence
  - drought
  - land contamination, e.g. Love Canal, USA
  - water contamination, e.g. Camelford
  - food chain contamination, e.g. BSE, E. coli/salmonella outbreaks.
- Other hazards:
  - serious untoward incidents, e.g. radiation leaks or maladministration of anti-cancer drugs
  - systematic laboratory error, e.g. failure of cancer screening processes
  - industrial action, e.g. UK Fire Service strikes in 2003
  - IT or other communications failure, e.g. Y2K
  - petrol crisis, e.g. UK fuel crisis in 2000
  - civil disorder or demonstrations, e.g. May Day demonstrations
  - threats or hoaxes, e.g. bomb threat
  - transport incidents, e.g. road traffic accidents.

Box 1.1 Kegworth disaster, 1989[1]

> In 1989 a plane carrying 126 passengers and crew crashed at Kegworth. Some 63% of those on board (82 people) survived. Transporting and treating them presented a considerable challenge for ambulance and acute hospitals which responded. The Leicestershire Ambulance Service had to provide 181 ambulance personnel, 14 officers and 75 vehicles, plus ambulance control and liaison staff. They treated and transported 82 seriously injured patients to hospital 76 within two and a half hours.
>
> Three receiving hospitals had to cope with this mass influx of patients, who between them sustained 191 fractures, as well as other serious injuries. Pressure on A&E casualty resuscitation, theatre and ITU was intense. This was all on a Sunday, when there was no routine work going on and both theatre space and staff were free. What would the consequences have been if Kegworth had happened on a busy weekday?

1.2.2 Disasters

Research scholars from around the world have been debating the meaning of the word 'disaster' for many years. Such debate has spawned many definitions, but all agree that disasters are usually sudden impact events that can cause disruption to society. Although definitions are agreed in the UK, it is important to recognise that the debate around the definition of a disaster continues internationally. Some of the definitions are outlined below.

Kreps (cited in Quarantelli 1998) suggests disasters are:

> ... non routine events in societies or their larger subsystems (e.g. regions, communities) that involve social disruption and physical harm. Among the key defining properties of such events are (1) length of forewarning, (2) magnitude of impact, (3) scope of impact, and (4) duration of impact.

Erikson (cited in Quarantelli 1998) suggests disasters:

> ... involve considerable harm to the physical and social environment; they happen suddenly or are socially defined as having reached one or more acute stages; and something can be done to mitigate their effects before or after they happen.

Hewitt (cited in Quarantelli 1998) defines disasters as:

> ... unmanaged phenomena. They are the unexpected, the unprecedented. They derive from natural processes of events that are highly uncertain. Unawareness and unreadiness are said to typify the condition of their human victims. Even the common use of the word [disaster] 'event' can reinforce the idea of a discrete unit in time in space. In the unofficial euphemism for disasters in North America, they are 'unscheduled events'.

1.3 Public health context of major incidents

A public health incident is any event that presents a serious threat or potential threat to the health of the population or local community.[2] When this threat is severe or imminent, then the incident may become an emergency (Nicols 2003).

Public health incidents may include: outbreaks of infectious disease (e.g. salmonella, legionella, E. coli); epidemics or pandemics (SARS); acute chemical incidents like water contamination or chemical spills; chronic chemical incidents like land contamination; or a deliberate release chemical, biological, radiological and nuclear (CBRN) incident (see Chapter 10).

Box 1.2 Lanarkshire E.coli outbreak, 1996

On 22 November [1996], the Public Health Department of Lanarkshire Health Board became aware of several cases of E. coli [infection] in the central belt of Scotland. An outbreak control team was formed the next day to manage and control the tide of infection that peaked at more than 40 new cases a day. There were 1,000 cases altogether. The incident placed substantial pressures on local health resources. Tests on 969 people had to be carried out, and 127 people were admitted to hospital.

Despite most major incidents being sudden onset events, they can also arise in other ways, as illustrated below.

- **Big bang** – sudden emergency (e.g. train crash, explosion): immediately recognisable; quick development; the majority of casualties appear early on; it is often more easy to predict the course of events and estimate the scale of the incident.

- **Rising tide** – the problem creeps up gradually, such as occurs in a developing infectious disease epidemic or a winter bed availability crisis. There is no clear starting point for the major incident, and the point at which an outbreak becomes major may only be clear in retrospect.

Box 1.3 Influenza pandemic

Influenza pandemics have occurred at intervals varying between 11 and 42 years. In 1957, the Asian flu took six to seven months, from first being isolated in China, [before it] peaked [with] the epidemic in the UK, where there were an estimated 9 million cases. The most recent pandemic started in Hong Kong in July 1968. There was a relatively small outbreak in the UK in the winter of 1968–69, with a sharp epidemic in January 1970.

- **Cloud on horizon** – an incident in one place may affect others following the incident. Preparatory action is needed in response to an evolving threat elsewhere, even perhaps overseas, such as a major chemical or nuclear release, a dangerous epidemic or a war.

Box 1.4 Chernobyl, Ukraine, 1986

Two huge explosions destroyed a nuclear power station:

- 31 people died immediately and 135,000 were permanently evacuated.
- [As a result] radioactive fallout spread all over Europe.
- Several days elapsed before the full environmental implications and public concern in the UK were fully appreciated and the health services and other agencies [were] fully mobilised in response to the risks.

Often the recognition of a public health incident is due to the recognition of an unusual pattern of events or diagnosis, particularly in a rising-tide situation. Half the battle can be the recognition that something abnormal has occurred/is occurring and that awareness is raised to the possibilities that immediate action needs to be taken.

For reference to mass casualty incidents, refer to Chapter 10.

1.4 The disaster cycle

The process of dealing with disaster – from prevention to preparedness, and response to recovery – is known as the disaster cycle (the phases may also be known as Reduction, Readiness, Response and Recovery). Figure 1.1 graphically explains the process. It is an open-ended process, one that can take from as little as a few days to many months or even years. The importance of each phase in the cycle is highlighted below.

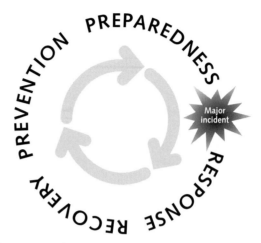

Figure 1.1 The disaster cycle

1.4.1 Prevention

Certain kinds of activity carry known risks and are subject to legal requirements for adopting prevention measures which aim to eliminate, isolate or reduce those risks as far as is reasonably practicable (Cabinet Office 2003).

Major incident management should seek to identify hazards in the local area by collaborating and liaising with partner agencies to ensure your organisation is aware of the risks in the community, and also in order to identify threats to your organisation. It may then be possible to work with partner agencies to prevent or minimise the impact of such hazards.

1.4.2 Preparedness

Preparation involves planning, training and exercising. Plans must provide the basis for an effective integrated response to major emergencies, whether they arise from known hazards or unforeseen events. A plan should provide a prepared and agreed framework within which organisations and individuals can work in a concerted manner. They are then in a better position to solve problems when they occur. There needs to be clear ownership of the plans and commitment to them from senior management (Cabinet Office 2003).

The preparedness phase – the period before the incident happens – involves setting up an efficient system for emergency response and remedial action influenced by the experience from previous incidents or training sessions. During this stage decisions can be made by consensus (Fairman et al. 2001).

1.4.3 Response

With sudden impact emergencies (explosions, major transport accidents, riots) the initial response is normally provided by the statutory emergency services and, as necessary, by the appropriate local authorities and possibly voluntary organisations. Experience of slower onset or less localised emergencies or crises (BSE, the fuel protests of 2000, foot and mouth disease) shows that other organisations may well face the brunt even in the early stages of a major emergency (Cabinet Office 2003).

The response stage commences once an incident has been recognised and lasts as long as rapid interventions are conducted. It is characterised by pressure of time, rapid decision making (preferably according to a prearranged chain of command) and emergency responders' attempts to comply with prepared plans and arrangements (Irwin et al. 1999).

1.4.4 Recovery

Recovery management encompasses the physical, social, psychological, political and financial consequences of an emergency. Anticipation of consequences and appropriate recovery planning must start right from the beginning of any response. Organisations and communities need to plan, manage and undertake those activities that will provide as rapid a return to normality as possible – for both the community and responders. Lessons from the past emphasise the need to involve the community fully in its own recovery. The promotion and support of self-help activities are important considerations (Home Office 2003).

The recovery phase lasts as long as the effects of the incident can be expected to persist. Generally, more time is available to make decisions than in the response phase. However, public and political pressure may place time constraints on the remediation action. Legal action could be involved and questions of recovery of costs during an incident may be important. Once the response phase is over, victims start the process of coping with repercussions of the incident and communities and the media tend to return to their usual activities and lose interest in the incident and its consequences (Fairman et al. 2001).

Recovery can be described as the coordinated efforts and processes to effect the immediate, medium- and long-term holistic regeneration of a community following a disaster (MCDEM 2005).

1.5 Integrated arrangements for emergency management

Disasters have a variety of effects on society and the environment, and thus demand a combined and coordinated response, linking the expertise and resources of the emergency services and the local authorities, supplemented, as appropriate, by other organisations.

The underlying aim of integrating the arrangements for emergency management is the development of flexible plans which should enable any organisation to deal effectively with a major or minor emergency, whether foreseen or unforeseen.[3]

Integration of emergency management arrangements embraces a number of concepts, some of which overlap. These are:

(a) Firstly, that the principal emphasis in the development of any plan must be on the response to the incident and not the cause of the incident. Planning arrangements for a range of emergencies, whether caused naturally or resulting from technical failure, or by a deliberate act of terrorism, must be integrated. The plan has to be flexible; it has to work on a bank holiday weekend or in freezing weather conditions, and at any location. It will need to be tested against specific scenarios.

(b) Secondly, emergency management arrangements should be integrated into an organisation's everyday working structure. Emergency plans must build on routine arrangements and it is therefore essential for those who will be required to respond to any emergency to be involved in the planning process and subsequent exercises.

(c) Thirdly, the activities of different departments within an organisation should be integrated. The overall response to a crisis will invariably need input from a number of different departments. Effective planning must integrate these contributions and establish protocols in order to achieve an efficient and timely response to an incident. Not to be aware of the contribution which will need to be made by other sections within an organisation is a recipe for a muddled response.

(d) Fourthly, there is a vital need to coordinate arrangements with other authorities and organisations. Major disasters will almost always span boundaries, and indeed may spread. If the response is to be truly effective in meeting the needs of everyone caught up in the disaster, then all leaders of industry, commerce and the community have to be aware of the roles their organisations may be called upon to play and how they fit into the response as a whole (Home Office 2003).

1.6   Summary

This chapter has provided definitions of disaster and major incidents. It has identified the way in which disasters and major incidents can arise and examined the phases of the disaster cycle. Finally, it has given an introduction to and an overview of integrated emergency management.

1.7   Notes

1. The text of Boxes 1.1 to 1.4 is reproduced from the Department of Health (1998) document, *Planning for Major Incidents: The NHS Guidance*, with the kind permission of the Department of Health.

2. Section 1.3 of this chapter is reproduced from *Planning for Major Incidents: The NHS Guidance*, with the kind permission of the Department of Health.

3. Apart from the first paragraph, the text of section 1.5 is reproduced from *Dealing With Disaster* (2003), with the kind permission of Crown Copyright.

2

Emergency Management: the Legal Framework in the UK

Eve Coles and Jim Stuart-Black

2.1 Introduction

The legislation that governs the way major incidents are dealt with in the UK is varied, ranging from that which determines the response of local authorities on the one hand, to the way in which NHS Acute Trusts and Primary Care Trusts (PCTs) respond on the other. This chapter describes the legislation that determines why we plan for major incidents, and includes the following areas:

- Civil Contingencies Act 2004
- regulations relating to Acute Trusts and PCTs
- health and safety at work
- duty of care
- human rights
- local authority response.

2.2 Civil Contingencies Act 2004

Increasing awareness of the diverse and frequently complex risks facing society, coupled with major emergencies and terrorist attacks, indicated that historical emergency legislation, such as the 1920 Emergency Powers Act and the 1948 Civil Defence Act, is no longer adequate – civil defence is no longer to be considered as a stand-alone activity. Following the floods and fuel crisis in 2000, the foot and mouth crisis of 2001, an extensive review of emergency planning arrangements, broad consultation and legislative review, the Civil Contingencies Act 2004 was drawn up and received Royal assent in November 2004. The Act was implemented in April 2005.

Whilst detailed examination of the Act is beyond the scope of this chapter, it is essential that all health organisations familiarise themselves with it, as it places a significant requirement upon the health sector. It is important to remember that it is an enabling Act paving the way for the establishment of regulations and statutory guidance. The Act may seem to lack specific detail, but the detail is in the regulations and guidance that have followed; these set the specific expectations for civil protection. The Act has increased legislated requirements upon a number of organisations classed as either Category 1 or Category 2 responders. (Health, except for Strategic Health Authorities, has been classified as Category 1.) Box 2.1 illustrates a limited number of brief summary comments; extra information is provided where relevant in the remainder of this handbook, and the Act and associated regulations and guidance are available for review on the UK Resilience website.

The Act sets out:

- a definition of the term 'emergency'
- the provision for identification of risks and the development of a community risk register

- a duty to plan for civil emergencies
- a duty for responders to share information
- a categorisation of responders
- a duty for first responders to have business continuity plans in place
- a duty for local authorities to provide advice and support to the business community
- a provision to declare a state of emergency on a regional basis
- a provision for warning and informing the public
- a provision for the appointment of regional coordinators
- a provision for the Minister of State to draw up a regulatory framework for dealing with emergencies.

Box 2.1 Health as a Category 1 responder

Health

5 A National Health Service Trust established under section 5 of the National Health Service and Community Care Act 1990 (c. 19) if, and in so far as, it has the function of providing:

(a) Ambulance Services

(b) hospital accommodation and services in relation to accidents and emergencies, or

(c) services in relation to public health in Wales.

6 An NHS foundation Trust (within the meaning of section 1 of the Health and Social Care (Community Health and Standards) Act 2003 (c. 43)) if, and in so far as, it has the function of providing hospital accommodation and services in relation to accidents and emergencies.

7 A Primary Care Trust established under section 16A of the National Health Service Act 1977 (c. 49).

8 A local health board established under section 16BA of the National Health Service Act 1977.

9 The Health Protection Agency (a special health authority established under section 11 of the National Health Service Act 1977).

10 A port health authority constituted under section 2 (4) of the Public Health (Control of Disease) Act 1984 (c. 22).

(Civil Contingencies Act 2004: 21)

Amongst other functions, Category 1 responders are required to:

- assess, plan and advise as required
- cooperate in local resilience forums
- carry out risk assessments from time to time
- collaborate in maintaining a community risk register(s)
- share information as required
- maintain certain plans
- carry out training
- respond as required.

All Category 1 responders have until November 2005 to comply with the terms of the Act.

2.3 Regulations relating to Acute Trusts and PCTs

The need for hospitals to plan for major incidents was first recognised in the National Health Service Act 1977. The Act required all hospitals with accident and emergency departments (now Acute Trusts) to have in place an emergency plan that could be operationalised in the event of a major incident occurring.

PCT Functions (Amendment) Regulations 2002 require PCTs to carry out planning for major incidents under sections 2–5 of the National Health Act 1977. Chief Executives of PCTs have responsibility for ensuring that plans and arrangements are in place for their own PCT; these should also include collaborative arrangements with neighbouring NHS organisations and partner agencies. Nominated lead PCTs perform the coordination function previously carried out by Health Authorities (Court 2002).

2.4 Health and safety legislation

The Health and Safety Executive (HSE) is the enforcing authority for health and safety law in relation to the health services.[1] The HSE will be involved in any criminal investigation of a health authority's or Trust's role in a major incident, but the police would lead the investigation of any possible manslaughter case. The main focus for the HSE is the cause of the incident, but it can, and does, consider the role of the emergency services and the health service.

As well as the general duties under the Health and Safety at Work Act 1974, there is a set of regulations that are relevant to major incident planning. The Management of Health and Safety at Work Regulations 1999 (S.I. 1999/3242 – ISBN 0110856252) require employers to:

- assess risks to their employees while at work, and any risks to others which arise from the course of their undertaking

- identify the measures that need to be taken to control those risks

- have adequate written arrangements for planning, organising, control, monitoring and review of those measures.

The regulations specifically address procedures for dealing with serious and imminent danger and contact with external services, particularly medical care and rescue work.

The Regulations should be read in conjunction with *Management of Health and Safety at Work – Approved Code of Practice and Guidance* – ISBN 0717624889.

Health Authorities and Trusts must be aware of the relevant health and safety legislation and that the Health and Safety Executive has wide powers to investigate accidents.

The Health and Safety at Work Act 1974 is the principal Act concerning all aspects of health and safety at work. It places a duty on employers to ensure, so far as is reasonably practicable, the health, safety and welfare at work of all employees, persons contracted to them and members of the public (Eagles et al. 2003).

Regulations drawn up under the Act of major relevance for those involved with managing chemical incidents are:

- **Control of Major Accident Hazards Regulations 1999** (COMAH), which apply to establishments where specified dangerous substances are kept in specified quantities

- **Chemical Hazard Information and Packaging Regulations 1994** (CHIP), which aim to protect people and the environment from the detrimental effect of chemicals by means of labelling and the provision of safety data sheets

- **Control of Substances Hazardous to Health Regulations 1994** (COSHH), which apply to toxic, harmful, corrosive or irritant substances defined in the CHIP regulations and to all places of work

- **Notification of Installations Handling Hazardous Substances Regulations 1982** (NIHHS), which require operators of sites where certain specified quantities and types of materials are stored or handled to notify details to the HSE

- **Control of Asbestos in the Air Regulations 1990** and **Control of Asbestos at Work Regulations 1987**, which apply to the air pollution aspects of asbestos and occupational exposure to asbestos respectively

- **Control of Lead at Work Act 1998** (CLAW), which requires employers to assess the occupational exposure risks from lead and adopt steps to prevent or minimise such exposure.

Hazardous installations

The Control of Major Accident Hazards Regulations 1999 (COMAH) require the operators of every establishment covered by the regulations to discharge a number of obligations, including notifying and keeping informed 'the competent authority', which in England and Wales are the HSE and the Environment Agency jointly.

The obligations under COMAH of particular relevance to Acute Trusts and PCTs, and the management of chemical incidents, relate to the preparation of on-site and off-site emergency plans. COMAH Regulation 9 requires operators to produce an 'on-site emergency plan', which should be adequate to deal with the on-site consequences of possible major accidents and provide assistance with mitigatory action. Regulation 9(3)(d) requires the operator to consult the appropriate Acute Trust/PCT on the preparation of the on-site emergency plan. This is an amendment to the 1999 document, which, following consultation with the health sector and the associated guidance, states:

> Health agencies should also be consulted, as they will have to deal with any injuries which arise and [are] responsible for ensuring that satisfactory arrangements are in place for handling the health-care aspects of the response to a major accident. This will include ensuring that arrangements are in place with acute hospital trusts and health agencies for the treatment of any casualties that may arise. It will also include determining, where appropriate, the most suitable holding locations for supplies of up-to-date stocks of antidotes.

Regulation 10 also states that each local authority must have an off-site emergency plan for each relevant establishment in its area. In preparing the off-site emergency plan, the local authority must consult the Acute Trust/PCT for the area. Under Regulation 11 emergency plans must be reviewed and tested from time to time, and under Regulation 12 an emergency plan (whether on- or off-site) must be put into effect when there is a major accident or an uncontrolled event which could reasonably be expected to lead to a major accident.

2.5   Duty of care

A duty of care is an obligation to conduct an activity in a safe manner. In the context of emergency planning, this could include the duty of an Ambulance Trust to arrive on the scene within a certain period of time, or the duty of an Acute Trust to have a system in place for prioritising the treatment of the more seriously injured.

The common law can establish a duty of care through many different situations, including written contract, oral representations, or custom and practice.

It is essential that there is:

- A relationship of proximity between the parties, i.e. there has to be established an actual or apparent relationship between the parties. This is sometimes referred to as 'the neighbour principle'.
- Foreseeability, i.e. the harm caused could reasonably be expected to have happened as a consequence of negligence.

The breach of the duty of care

A breach of duty of care depends upon the facts of each case. Examples could include:

- not having an emergency plan
- failing to implement an emergency plan properly
- failing to respond to a major incident in reasonable time
- failing to comply with published guidelines and directions
- having insufficient resources to deal with a major incident, and
- failing to justify that insufficiency.

The breach must cause actionable damage

A breach must manifest itself in some way. The classic instance would be physical injury or exacerbated physical injury which has resulted in loss. The emphasis of the law is on physical injury. Purely economic loss (loss not consequent on physical damage) is usually irrecoverable in the courts.[2]

For advice relating to liability or insurance issues, please refer to *Planning for Major Incidents: The NHS Guidance*, or seek advice from the Department of Health.

2.6 Human rights

The Human Rights Act 1998 came into effect on 2 October 2000, and effectively incorporates the European Convention on Human Rights (ECHR) into English law. Its primary application is between individuals and public authorities, including health protection agencies and hospital trusts as well as local authorities. Section 6(1) states that '(i)t is unlawful for a public authority to act in a way which is incompatible with a Convention right', and Section 6(6) makes clear that 'an "act" includes a failure to act'. Section 7 provides for an individual who claims that a public authority has acted or proposes to act in a way that is incompatible with his or her convention rights, to bring proceedings in court. Therefore, an individual or a company may bring proceedings against any health agency, claiming that it has acted or failed to act, or is about to do so, in a way which is incompatible with his, her or its convention rights.

Health authorities and local authorities are required to consider human rights when carrying out their duties as described, for example, by Integrated Pollution Prevention and Control (IPPC) and the COMAH Regulations. Article 2 of the ECHR states that '(e)veryone's right to life shall be protected by law.' The European Court of Human Rights has frequently held that this places on public authorities, including health authorities, a positive obligation to protect life.

Although under IPPC and COMAH the health agencies are not statutorily requested to respond, the Department of Health has now indicated that this is the case. Failure to respond, or the provision of inadequate or incorrect advice and comment by health agencies, could give rise to a claim under Sections 6 and 7 of the Human Rights Act if death, injury or even damage to property (under Article 8 of the ECHR), which could have been avoided, were suffered.

2.7 Local authority legislation

There are a number of different Acts of Parliament and regulations that govern the way local authorities respond to civil defence and emergencies. It is worth emphasising that until April 2005 the only compulsion on local authorities was to plan for civil defence.

The legislative framework that underpinned emergency planning in England and Wales was a patchwork of Acts, which began with the Civil Defence Act 1948 and developed through a series of ad hoc measures introduced over the last fifty years. The 1948 Act allowed the Home Secretary to introduce regulations affecting the functions of local authorities and their ability to deal with defence of the civil population 'against any form of hostile attack by a foreign power' (Tucker 1999). The Act also provided for a grant from central government to fund the civil defence activities of local authorities. However, this Act and some of the subsequent legislation has now been superseded by the Civil Contingencies Act 2004.

Various statues and regulations are still in force, including:

- **Local Government Act 1972**, which allows local authorities to spend money to 'avert, alleviate or eradicate' the effects caused by disasters (Turney 1990).

- **Control of Major Accident Hazards Regulations 1999** (COMAH) (refer to section 2.4 for details).

- **The Radiation Emergencies (Preparedness and Public Information) Regulations 2001** (REPPIR), which impose a duty on fire and civil defence authorities, and county and unitary councils, to prepare plans to provide information to the public in the event of a 'radiation emergency'. Operators of sites in the UK liable to give rise to radiation emergencies (this could include all health agencies) have to provide information to the public and consult local authorities. Local authorities are responsible for information referring to radiation emergencies originating overseas (for example, Chernobyl) (Harthman 2002).

2.8 Summary

This chapter has summarised the law relating to emergency planning in England and Wales. With regard to the health service, it has covered regulations relating to Acute Trusts and PCTs, health and safety at work, major chemical sites (COMAH) and duty of care. Finally, it has covered the law relating to local authority emergency planning.

2.9 Notes

1. Section 2.4 is reproduced from Department of Health (1998), with the kind permission of the Department of Health.

2. This information is reproduced from Department of Health (1998), with the kind permission of the Department of Health.

3

Crisis Management and Organisational Learning

Eve Coles

3.1 Introduction

Over the last few years the National Health Service (NHS) has suffered from a number of prominent crises, including the BSE crisis and the E. coli outbreak in Scotland. As a result of these and other well-documented crises, the Chief Medical Officer (CMO) commissioned a panel of experts to investigate how the NHS might learn from its mistakes. Their published report, entitled *An Organisation with a Memory*, details how the NHS can identify lessons to be learned and embed these lessons within the organisation. Such concepts are of importance to health emergency planners, particularly in the event of a major incident or crisis (or even a training exercise) where the lessons identified need to be implemented as soon as possible after the event.

This chapter aims to give a brief overview of the importance of crisis management strategy and organisational learning. It includes sections on:

- crisis management
- organisational learning from crisis in the NHS
- barriers to organisational learning.

3.2 Crisis management

The term 'crisis' comes from the Greek *krinein*, meaning to decide, or a decisive moment or turning point. Other definitions include:

> ... a major, unpredictable event that has potentially negative results (Barton 1993, cited in Heath 1998)

> ... an event that brings, or has the potential for bringing, an organisation into disrepute and imperils its future profitability (Lerbinger 1997).

Crisis management is a strategic function of an organisation, and crisis management strategy is about asking how a crisis can be dealt with in a logical and orderly manner, to prevent it turning into a major incident. It will include:

- solving immediate problems or issues
- controlling and coordinating internal and external communications
- running the rest of the organisation in a controlled manner.

Crises differ from major incidents and disasters as they tend to generate doubt and suspicion about the reality and advent of danger.

Crises have a number of stages to them, which have been described by many researchers. Two examples are provided below.

Kash and Darling (1998) describe four distinct stages of a crisis:

- **Prodromal crisis stage:** a warning signal of the onset of crisis. Oblique and hard to detect.

- **Acute crisis stage** (impact): urgent action is required at this stage. However, any action taken will only limit damage, not prevent it.

- **Chronic crisis stage:** 'make or break' period in crisis development. Quick fixes may work short term, but long-term solutions need to be found.

- **Crisis resolution:** unresolved crisis can destroy an organisation, so action must be taken to root out causal factors and put them right.

In contrast, Mitroff and Pearson (1993) see five distinct phases:

- **Signal detection:** where organisational defences (if adequate) will pick up warning signals and deal with them (safety/reporting procedures).

- **Preparation/prevention:** risk assessment, plan writing and exercising.

- **Containment:** dealing with the incident to prevent escalation.

- **Recovery:** returning as near as possible to the pre-crisis state.

- **Learning:** debriefing and identifying the lessons to be learned and embedding them within the organisation.

A good crisis management strategy should include the following elements:

- **Reduction:** a good risk management programme that aims to reduce the threats to the organisation.

- **Readiness:** a well-written, tried and tested contingency plan that can be activated as soon as is needed.

- **Response:** well-trained personnel who are ready to respond at a moment's notice.

- **Recovery:** strategies in place to identify the lessons to be learned from the crisis, and the implementation of the learning process, thus allowing the organisation to recover from the incident as quickly as possible.

Implemented properly, these '**four Rs**' can lead to a fifth R, that of **resilience** to crisis. Understanding the full implications of crisis events helps an organisation to develop resilience.

3.3 Organisational learning from crisis in the NHS

Learning from crisis events[1] and applying this knowledge to future situations has two core aims:

- to reduce exposure to future crisis situations and their impacts

- to increase the psychological and organisational readiness of the organisation to respond to crisis situations and to recover from them when they cannot be avoided.

Research on learning from failures in health care is relatively sparse, yet the evidence from other areas of activity – and in particular from industry – reveals a rich seam of valuable knowledge about the nature of failure and of learning which is as relevant to health care as to any other area of human activity.

When things go wrong, whether in health care or in another environment, the response has often been an attempt to identify an individual or individuals who must carry the blame. The focus of incident analysis has tended to be on the events immediately surrounding an adverse event, and in particular on the human acts or omissions immediately preceding the event itself.

Organisational learning is a cyclical process, the key components of which can be described with reference to an approach which we have adapted from a model used by British Petroleum in the context of its work on knowledge management (Figure 3.1). Of necessity, this model greatly oversimplifies the process it depicts – omitting, for example, the important dimension of feedback 'short circuits' within the process – but it serves to illustrate the fundamental steps in a learning cycle.

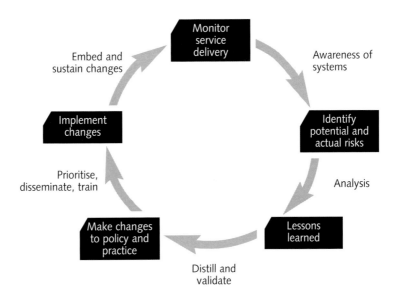

Figure 3.1 The learning cycle

The process does not differ, regardless of whether learning takes place before, during or after the event. The first half of the learning cycle essentially concerns the identification of learning opportunities and the development of sound solutions. Monitoring of service delivery activity – including adverse events and the experiences of others – provides a basis for asking questions about how improvements can be brought about and errors avoided. Some commentators have suggested that a key part of this process is 'sensemaking' – ensuring that individuals and organisations actually understand what the true nature of their experience is, so that it provides a sound basis for learning. It is far more difficult for effective learning to take place if the initial understanding of what has occurred is seriously flawed. In particular, it is important to consider experiences in the context of the various systems in place and the way these interact, because only in this way is it possible to come to sound conclusions about the nature of potential and actual risks faced.

Once potential and actual risks have been identified, they must be properly analysed to identify lessons for policy and practice. Lessons can be extracted from the pool of available information through analysis, but they then need to be distilled – to make sure that the essence of the learning points is properly captured – and their validity tested in theory or practice. Validation is important where ideas come from experience in other sectors or organisations – transferability is often possible but cannot be assumed – but it is also a key step in learning from experience within a team or an organisation. It is all too easy to reach a conclusion or draw a lesson which appears obvious, but which does not in fact stand up to testing. The initial assessment of the experience or diagnosis of the problem may be flawed, or the solution identified may not in practice address the issue effectively.

The second part of the learning process, once sound solutions have been derived, is to make sure that they are put into practice. Learning points need to be translated into practical policies and actions that can be implemented at the appropriate level. These practical changes then need to be prioritised, to provide a clear agenda for action, and then disseminated to the relevant audience. Training is a vital tool in ensuring that information on change is both disseminated and acted on.

Action to implement and apply improvements on the ground is an essential part of the learning process. Lessons can be 'learned' on one level, in that there is a strong awareness of what needs to change and why, but if there are barriers in place to the application of that learning in practice the active learning process will fail. However, to sustain long-term change, solutions also need to be firmly embedded into the culture and routine practice of the organisation. Only if change is successfully embedded in an organisation will it survive once the 'heat' is perceived to have gone out of a particular problem. If an organisation focuses intensively on a problem for a short period of time, but forgets about it when new priorities emerge or key personnel move on, effective learning has not taken place. As we have already observed, learning is not a one-off event, it is an ongoing dynamic.

Finally, continuous monitoring of changes and improvements in practice is an essential part of ongoing learning and improvement. All the evidence suggests that the latter stages in this learning process are critical in ensuring that organisational behaviour is actually changed as a result of the lessons drawn from adverse incidents, and that true 'learning' requires more than just the identification of valid lessons. But it is at the stages of implementation and embedding that the learning loop often seems to fracture.

A number of systems already exist in the NHS that can, to varying extents, be seen as mechanisms for learning from adverse health-care events, but collectively they have serious limitations. These NHS systems include:

- a number of local, regional and national incident reporting schemes
- ongoing national studies in specific areas of care, such as the four Confidential Inquiries
- systems, such as those for complaints and litigation, which are designed to investigate or respond to specific instances of poor-quality care
- periodic external studies and reviews (e.g. the Audit Commission's Value for Money studies)
- health and public health statistics, and
- a range of internal and external incident inquiries.

Some of these systems (such as the Confidential Inquiries and the national reporting system for incidents involving medical devices) achieve good coverage of very specific categories of event, and produce high-quality recommendations based on analysis of the information collected. Overall, though, coverage is patchy and there are many gaps.

Guidance on the reporting of adverse incidents in the NHS stretches back over 40 years, but there is still no standardised reporting system, nor indeed a standard definition of what should be reported.

Local risk-reporting systems, which should provide the bedrock for onward reporting to regional or national systems, are developing but similarly variable. Incident-reporting systems appear to be particularly poorly developed in primary care, and systematic reporting of 'near misses' (seen as an important early warning of serious problems) is almost non-existent across the NHS.

Systems vary, too, in the degree to which the information collected is subject to analysis with the aim of promoting learning. Information from the complaints system, and from health-care litigation in particular, appears to be greatly under-exploited as a learning resource. The NHS also secures variable value, both financially and in useful learning extracted, from the range of ad hoc incident investigations and inquiries undertaken every year. There is no single focal point for NHS information on adverse events, and at present it is spread across nearly 1,000 different organisations.

The NHS record in implementing the recommendations that emerge from these various systems is patchy. Too often lessons are identified, but true 'active' learning does not take place because the necessary changes are not properly embedded in practice. Though there is some good evidence of meaningful medium- and long-term change as a result of Confidential Inquiry recommendations, for example, this is rarely driven through into practice, and the onus for implementation and prioritisation is very much on local services. Take-up can tend to 'plateau' once changes have been implemented by those who are most naturally receptive to them, and there is some evidence that progress nationally can slip back if efforts are not sustained. Box 3.1 outlines two incidences of organisational failure to implement lessons learned.

Box 3.1 Case studies: failure to close the learning loop

Suicides by mental health inpatients

For some years it has been recognised that a major means of suicide among inpatients in mental health units is [by] hanging from curtain or shower rails. A paper drawing attention to this was first published in 1971. These events can be prevented fairly simply by fitting collapsible rails which give way under the weight of a person. The 1999 report of the National Confidential Inquiry into Suicides and Homicides by People with Mental Illness (Appleby 1999) concluded that hanging, and in particular hanging from non-collapsible structures such as bed and shower and curtain rails, is still the commonest method of suicide among mental health inpatients. A total of 81 mental health inpatients committed suicide on the ward by hanging in the two years to April 1998 – two thirds of all suicides which took place on the ward. On at least one occasion a collapsible curtain rail, which had given way, preventing a hanging, was incorrectly repaired. When another patient later attempted to hang himself from the same rail it failed to collapse and the patient died (Appleby 1999: 37).

Death due to incorrect urinary tract irrigation

A patient with urinary tract stones underwent a procedure, under anaesthetic, in which her upper urinary tract should have been washed out with a special fluid. In fact, plain water was used by mistake. The water affected the patient's bloodstream, and she suffered a fatal heart attack in the operating theatre. Despite details of the incident being circulated to all relevant hospitals, a second similar incident almost occurred within a few months in a hospital only 30 miles away. Fortunately, in this case the mistake was spotted before the fluid could be administered, and no harm came to the patient. The surgeon involved pointed out that, at a distance, the bags of different irrigating fluids looked identical (Department of Health 1998).

These NHS case studies are good examples of the phenomenon of 'passive' learning: valid lessons have been drawn from experience, but they have not been fully implemented. By contrast, 'active' learning involves both drawing valid conclusions and putting them into practice. It is only through active learning that the benefits of experience are actually realised. Some NHS examples of 'active learning' – where effective changes in practice do appear to have been made to prevent particular problems recurring – are provided by the 'Back to Sleep' campaign to reduce cot deaths.

Box 3.2 The 'Back to Sleep' campaign – active learning in the NHS saved the lives of 3,000 babies

In the 1970s and 1980s, advice given to new parents by health-care professionals was that babies should be placed in their cots on their fronts. [In this way] it was reasoned that if a baby regurgitated milk, choking was less likely [to occur] than if the baby were lying on its back. Research from several countries, confirmed by work from Bristol published in 1990, found that babies placed on their backs had a lower incidence of 'cot death'. An expert group, convened by the then Chief Medical Officer in October 1991, reviewed this and further evidence from Bristol, where the cot death rate had fallen after health-care professionals started encouraging mothers to avoid prone sleeping positions in 1989. As a result, from December 1991 the Department of Health and the media ran a campaign to educate parents (the 'Back to Sleep' campaign). Cot deaths have halved in the years since the campaign. This is an example of rapid, active learning in the NHS, which led to the saving of over 3,000 babies' lives in the six years up to 1998 (Department of Health 1998).

In general, experience in the NHS and in other organisations suggests that individuals may learn from their mistakes, but those around them often fail to do so. Individuals may learn because mistakes cause them emotional pain, even if they go unnoticed by others. In some cases, of course, individuals may refrain from hearing key messages as a kind of personal 'defence mechanism' – this is partly a personality feature, though people can be taught to apportion responsibility more reasonably.

3.4 Barriers to organisational learning

Research has shown that it is possible to identify a number of different barriers that conspire to prevent learning in organisations. Smith and Elliott (2000) have suggested a number of barriers to learning, as set out in Table 3.1.

Many of the barriers listed are consequent on the fundamental problems associated with communication and core beliefs:

- A central element of the problem consists of those values and assumptions which are thought to be of importance in helping to develop a crisis-prone culture within organisations. These values and assumptions can be seen to be a central factor in inhibiting learning.

Table 3.1 Barriers to learning (Smith and Elliott 2000)

- Rigidity of core beliefs, values and assumptions.
- Ineffective communication and information difficulties.
- Lack of corporate responsibility.
- Incrementalist approach to problem solving (failure to deal with emergence).
- Reconstruction of event narrative and the projection of blame.
- Focus on single loop learning and a failure to address the manner of decision making.
- Peripheral inquiry and the influence of decoy phenomenon.
- Centrality of expertise, denial and the disregard of outsiders.
- Cognitive narrowing and event fixation (reductionist approach).
- Maladaption, threat minimisation and environmental shifts.

A second, important barrier is that of communication:

- The language used to communicate the nature of the risk is couched within the language of experts, which, in turn, is responsible for the concentration of experts within the decision-making process. This language is often impenetrable by local publics and thereby prevents or hinders effective discourse between those engaged in debates.

- The idea that certain groups cannot enter the debate because they have no recognised expertise in the field is often used to prevent them from entering into debates on risk that allow for a construction of cultural differences between expert and non-expert groups.

Other barriers include:

- **Scant attention to other events and near misses:** emphasises the value of 'hindsight'; not identifying the lessons to be learned from other disasters or near misses can allow the same mistakes to happen again and again.

- **Lack of corporate responsibility:** where the organisation and particularly those in control refuse to take ownership of responsibility for their actions.

- **Scapegoating:** looking for someone or something else to blame.

- **Mistrust (blameism):** a predominant organisational culture where admitting mistakes means being held accountable.

Therefore the resilience of an organisation is improved when:

- the likelihood of mistakes happening is accepted
- there is an acceptance of diversity and cooperation within the organisation/community
- there is an acceptance that technology can solve some crises but not all
- each person takes responsibility for themselves and their own actions.

A proactive approach to crisis management and an adoption of crisis-prepared strategies will lead to:

- safer organisational structures and facilities
- fewer workplace injuries and non-productive time
- an improved market position when less well-prepared organisations suffer similar crises
- confidence in the organisation, which can have spin-offs in terms of higher productivity and more satisfied employees or members of a community.

3.5 Summary

This chapter provided a brief overview of concepts related to crisis management and organisational learning. The chapter included sections on crisis management, organisational learning from crisis in the NHS, and barriers to organisational learning, which can be applied to an emergency management context to understand the process of organisational change.

3.6 Notes

1. Section 3.3 is reproduced from the Department of Health publication (2002a) *An Organisation with a Memory*, with the kind permission of the Department of Health.

4

Hazard Identification and Risk Assessment

Jim Stuart-Black

4.1 Introduction

Fundamental to the planning process is an understanding of what you are planning for – are you planning for a one-off catastrophic incident, a multiple vehicle traffic accident or a fire within a hospital wing? Without knowing the answer to these questions, the planning process is largely redundant. The process of identifying and quantifying hazards, and the associated risks threatening your organisation and working practices, is the first step to managing major incidents both in terms of response and, perhaps more critically, in terms of prevention.

Within any organisation, accurate risk and hazard assessment and subsequent planning initiatives will assist in reducing both tangible and intangible losses. Tangible losses include the loss of life, reduction in staff availability, or loss of buildings or equipment. Intangible losses, whilst slightly harder to identify and subsequently manage, will include loss of reputation through poor incident management or staffing practices. Before risks can be effectively planned for, it is necessary to identify and quantify them through a process of hazard identification and risk assessment.

The Civil Contingencies Act places a statutory duty on all Category 1 responders (see section 2.2) to undertake risk assessments. Based on the Australia/New Zealand Risk Management framework (4360:1999/2004), the assessment must recognise the risk of an emergency directly within or threatening the geographical area for which the responder is responsible.

Historically, many have felt that hazard identification and risk assessments were highly complicated and therefore best left to 'specialists'. Unfortunately, this has meant that the processes have not necessarily had the full participation of all members of the health service. However, the Act and subsequent regulations now ensure that health has a key role to play in the process. This chapter aims to provide a clear introduction to the hazard identification and risk assessment process, in order to ensure that the expertise and experience of all health service employees are utilised within this process, thus ensuring that it becomes an embedded practice.

4.2 Definitions

4.2.1 Hazard

A 'hazard' is anything that is 'a source of potential harm or a situation with the potential to cause loss' (Emergency Management Australia 2000). Critical to the hazard identification process is an understanding that hazards are not 'events' in their own right; rather, they represent the 'potential for an event' (World Health Organisation 1996).

4.2.2 Hazard identification

This is the term used for gathering information about hazards – potential sources of harm/loss within a definable area. The process of identifying hazards is not an exact science and may be done using either an arithmetic process or through simple discussion and research.

4.2.3 Risk

There are a number of different definitions of risk. For the purpose of this chapter, risk will be defined as 'the likelihood of an identified hazard causing harm'.

4.2.4 Risk assessment

The process of identifying and quantifying risks can be done in a number of ways. For the purpose of this chapter, the risk assessment process will be detailed in terms of frequency and severity. More detail on the assessment process is given later on in this chapter.

4.2.5 Vulnerability

Vulnerability defines the 'susceptibility and resilience' (Emergency Management Australia 2000: 4) to identified hazards of a group of individuals, communities, buildings or working practices. The term 'susceptibility' is used to detail the features of a particular working practice or group of people, etc. that allow a hazard to pose potential harm. (Note: it is not suggested that people or organisations willingly expose themselves to these sources of harm.) Resilience is the ability of an organisation or working practice, etc. to prepare for, respond to and recover from the likely impact of a hazard and associated risks.

> **RISK: Likelihood of an identified hazard causing harm.**
>
> **HAZARD: Source of potential harm or potential loss.**
>
> **VULNERABILITY: Susceptibility and resilience.**

4.3 Why conduct a risk assessment?

The risk assessment will identify risks facing an organisation and serve as a means to rank them according to their severity. Having identified the risks facing an organisation, department or an individual event, managers and staff will be able to take actions to reduce, remove or manage the risks.

4.4 Perception and context

The process of identifying and quantifying both risks and hazards is frequently a subjective process, as all individuals will see things differently. Owing to these differences, it is important to understand the issues surrounding perception. Both the risk assessment and hazard identification processes should include a number of stakeholders (the number and origin of these stakeholders will vary); clearly, what will be a hazard in the eyes of one may not be in the eyes of another. Examples of stakeholders within the health economy will include patients, clinicians, managers, the public and, in the case of private hospitals, shareholders.

Understanding the variations in risk and hazard perception will assist in establishing the context of the assessment process; this will set the scope and limitations of the risk assessment and the criteria against which risk should be judged. It should decide whether the assessment will be conducted at a strategic or operational level, what legal responsibilities the organisation has, exactly what will be included in the risk/hazard assessment, and what level of risk/hazard is considered to be:

- tolerable (not requiring action)
- significant (requiring action as soon as possible)
- critical (not acceptable and requiring immediate action).

4.5　The risk assessment process

As a Category 1 responder, health is required to contribute to the development of a community risk register (CRR). Rather than developing its assessment in isolation, health is encouraged to participate in collaborative workshops with other Category 1 responders within its area. Once developed, responders are required to ensure that their assessment is published – notable exceptions to this requirement are commercially sensitive or security-related risks.

There are many different approaches to assessing risk, but ultimately *it is essential to consider any existing risk assessment criteria currently utilised within your own organisation to ensure compliance with organisational standards.* This chapter provides a broad overview of some of the generic components to be undertaken as part of a risk assessment process; these are summarised in Figure 4.1.

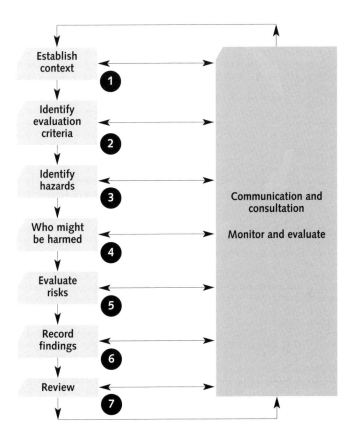

Figure 4.1 Generic risk management framework (adapted from MCDEM 2002)

Step 1: Establish the context ❶

Establishing the context serves to define the parts of the world we own and/or can influence. The process also serves to assist in clarifying our responsibilities. Whilst individual and organisational responsibilities will vary across the country, there will be broad similarities in terms of the commitment to your Local Resilience Forum and the development of a community risk register in accordance with the draft regulations supporting the Civil Contingencies Act 2004. Similarly, all health organisations have financial, operational, social, cultural and legal responsibilities.

Possible steps to assist with defining context may include:

- identifying internal and external stakeholders and their objectives
- describing the local physical environment
- identifying applicable strategic plans, reports and legal, social and cultural obligations.

Step 2: Identify risk evaluation criteria ❷

Risk evaluation criteria assist in determining whether or not a risk should be treated and, if so, the strategy for doing so. The risk evaluation criteria should be based upon real world 'objective' constraints that may be placed upon your risk evaluation process. Risk evaluation criteria might include the specification of acceptable and/or unacceptable risks, or the identification of methods/processes for the assessment of the cost/benefit ratio for treating risks.

Step 3: Identify the hazards ❸

Hazard identification should be done by a panel of stakeholders – consider the issues surrounding perception as discussed in section 4.4. The broad make up of the assessing panel will ensure that a diverse range of hazards is identified; it is suggested that the assessing panel will most likely be part of the existing emergency planning team within your organisation. To keep the process straightforward, it is recommended that a simple table be drawn up and that all members of the panel simply list perceived hazards. Once the list has been created, plainly prioritise, as a group, an order of magnitude, i.e. low, medium or high.

Step 4: Decide who might be harmed and how ❹

Having generated a comprehensive list of hazards that are perceived to be sources of potential harm to your organisation or operational practices, it is now necessary to decide what, if anything, is vulnerable to the identified hazards.

In section 4.2.5, vulnerability was defined in reference to susceptibility and resilience in terms of an individual, organisation, community, property, working practice and so on. In deciding who might be harmed and how, it is now possible to develop a form of quantification to build up a more detailed understanding of the 'risks' (refer to definitions in section 4.2.5) posed by the hazards defined through Step 1.

Working within a group, develop a simple chart on a large sheet of paper, and collectively develop a picture of risks associated with each identified hazard; it is likely that many of the hazards will be associated with multiple risks. For example, a fire is a hazard to which people and property are vulnerable – fire presents the risk of burns, damage to property, financial loss and, if poorly managed, damage to reputation.

This analogy serves as a good example of the benefit of looking outside the box in a holistic manner and examining risks in terms of both tangible and intangible consequences. Remember: anything and anyone can be vulnerable – hazard identification and risk assessment are not just about people.

Step 5: Evaluate the risks and decide whether the existing precautions are adequate or whether more should be done ❺

Assessing risk within a modular framework will make the process of evaluation far simpler. Models provide a logical framework in which to assess the risks. They can be quantitative or qualitative. Qualitative models, which require less specialist training, are often as effective as more complex quantitative models and benefit from being more accessible to a greater number of users. It is important to ensure that the model selected is both appropriate for the task and accessible to all those who will have to use and interpret its results.

Owing to the wide range of risk assessment models available, a model taken from the Department of Health has been chosen and adapted for this handbook. The model chosen is easy to use and provides succinct and accessible results. It has two variables that are typically used to judge the level of risk: 1) the frequency of a risk occurring; and 2) the severity of its impact. By applying common assessment criteria to assess frequency and severity, it is possible to judge different risks by a universal standard.

To begin with, the risks identified from hazards should be categorised in terms of frequency and severity. Table 4.1 provides an example of how frequency and severity can be categorised.

Table 4.1 Frequency and severity (Department of Health 1992)

Frequency	Low	Rare and unpredictable
	Medium	Occasional, but too often to ignore
	High	Often and expected
Severity	Low	Inconvenient; cost within operating budget
	Medium	Major disruption; activity/income reduced
	High	Catastrophic/financial ruin

Having categorised the risks in terms of severity and frequency, it is now possible to develop a simple matrix, which will enable the planning group to assess the level of identified risks and rank them accordingly. An example of such a matrix is shown in Table 4.2. In this example, minor risks would be tolerable, requiring no action, whereas significant risks would require action as soon as possible, and critical risks would be deemed not acceptable and thus require immediate action.

Table 4.2 Risk assessment decision-making matrix (adapted from Department of Health 1992)

		Severity		
		Low	Medium	High
Frequency	Low	Minor risk	Minor risk	Significant risk
	Medium	Minor risk	Significant risk	Critical risk
	High	Significant risk	Critical risk	Critical risk

Step 6: Record your findings ❻

Hazard identification and risk assessments are iterative processes: they require continuity to allow comparison of new assessments with previous ones. To assist in recording changes, organisations need to develop standardised forms and processes that meet their individual requirements.

By its very nature the consideration of risk involves uncertainties, and whilst the best sources of data should be used when evaluating risk, where information is incomplete or missing it may be necessary to make subjective judgements and assumptions. When this is the case, it is important to document the fact and place a level of confidence on the judgement or assumption. During the evaluation process, the risk posed by a hazard can then be reviewed and updated according to more up-to-date information.

Step 7: Review your assessment and revise it if necessary to ensure it is adequately done ❼

Risk managers will use risk assessments to design risk reduction strategies. Once these strategies have been identified, the risk assessment process should be repeated to ensure that the suggested actions would reduce the risk to an acceptable level.

Few risks remain static: new hazards appear, the vulnerability of organisations changes as they develop, and the perceptions of stakeholders alter to reflect environmental changes. The risk assessment process must be an ongoing one, and thus it requires continuous monitoring and evaluation. The entire risk assessment process should be subject to regular review, but it must also be repeated when new hazards are identified and when a change in the organisation means that its vulnerability to the hazards is altered. Additionally, accidents and 'near misses' should trigger a review of the risk assessment.

Box 4.1 Example of an Acute Trust risk assessment

Fire Brigade industrial action – risk assessment

In mid-August 2002, the Fire Brigade announced that it was planning industrial action in response to the rejection of a new pay deal by the government. The Chief Executive Bulletin, covering the week 9–15 August, subsequently asked all NHS trusts to review their fire risk assessments, plans and contingency arrangements.

In response, the Whittington Hospital in north London applied some very simple principles of risk management. In the first instance, trust directors, the Health and Safety Adviser and Emergency Planning Liaison Officer (EPLO) met in order to:

- **identify the risks** to the hospital in terms of the risks to patients, staff and buildings
- look at ways to **remove or minimise risks** wherever possible
- **review emergency plans** in light of the above.

Below is a summary of the actions taken by the Whittington Hospital to mitigate risks where possible, and plan the response to those risks that remained.

Identify risks

It was of immediate concern that, in the event of an emergency to which the Fire Brigade would normally respond, the hospital would be left with a service which was limited by the relatively slow and poorly equipped Green Goddess fire-fighting appliances manned by the army.

- Health and Safety Adviser to discuss arrangements with the local fire authority regarding appropriate measures to be taken during the period of industrial action.
- Service Manager – Medicine to discuss the same issues with Health Emergency Planning Advisers.

Remove or minimise risks

Efforts to reduce the number of false alarms were increased. Contractors' activities were reviewed, and toasters on wards and in other departments were removed. In the event of the army needing to attend an incident at the Whittington, we took action to compensate for their lack of local knowledge about the hospital site. It was decided that the fire hydrants would be repainted yellow, and the Security Officer, who would meet an appliance at the front entrance to the hospital, was provided with a high-visibility jacket. Simple site maps and briefing sheets were placed in the Silver on-call folder and given to security staff.

Planning for an emergency

Raising the profile of existing plans

Normal fire prevention measures were assigned to a higher profile, including:

- line managers undertaking daily inspections of the workplace
- improving staff awareness and maintaining general housekeeping standards
  o the number of security patrols was increased, both to unoccupied areas and out of hours.

Special arrangements

- The trust's fire emergency response systems should ensure a rapid provision of 30 staff to assist in the first emergency phase of any fire evacuation scenario. During the period of industrial action, portering staff were included in this team to assist with any first aid fire fighting, fetching/carrying fire extinguishers or assisting in any evacuation as necessary.
- Following any immediate evacuation as above, the major incident call out system would then be initiated to assist with any subsequent moves between wards and to ensure adequate continuation of patient care. In addition, a member of the Gold team would have been expected to attend and work with the Silver on-call team to liaise with London Ambulance Service (LAS)/Emergency Bed Service (EBS) and local hospitals to transfer patients as necessary.
- In order to assist with any emergency power, natural gas, medical gas or other service shutdowns, arrangements were made for an estates engineer to maintain a 24-hour on-site presence during the period of industrial action.

Activation of emergency plans

The activation of a fire alarm in a patient-critical area was to result in an immediate 999 call from switchboard. The activation of an alarm in other areas was to be investigated by a security officer and would only result in a 999 call if smoke or fire were found.

Stand down

Security officers were to ensure that once a false alarm had been confirmed, switchboard staff were immediately advised to cancel the 999 call rapidly.

The Silver bleep holder was to assume sole responsibility for authorising the resetting of fire alarms on the advice of the security officers at the scene. If there was any doubt at all, then the alarm was not to be reset.

Reporting

Throughout the strikes, LAS HQ was coordinating all 999 calls normally received by the Fire Brigade. Any fire or chemical related incidents resulting in a 999 call needed to be reported to them as soon as possible after the event, via an incident form sent to a dedicated fax line.

During the fire strikes, the Whittington made two such reports. In both cases, the calls were false alarms, and the 999 calls were cancelled before the Green Goddesses arrived at the hospital.

The fire-strike contingency plans were devised by trust directors, the Health and Safety Adviser and EPLO.

Mark Avery
Service Manager – Medicine and Clinical Services
Emergency Planning Liaison Officer (EPLO)

4.6 Summary

The processes of hazard identification and risk assessment have traditionally been steeped in a degree of mystery, suggesting that only the 'specialists' can undertake them. This chapter has shown that whilst it is possible to apply a mathematical approach, discussion and common sense will often serve as an equally accurate approach. Effective hazard identification and, in turn, effective risk assessments are fundamental to the planning process – so much so that if plans have been written and developed without this solid foundation, what validity they will have, if any, is questionable. It is of paramount importance to ensure that the planning process is not done in isolation or considered in terms of just tangible consequences – reputation is everything and intangible losses can be just as devastating.

5

Planning for Major Incidents

Les Moseley

5.1 Introduction

Emergency plans can take many different forms. They may be in paper or electronic format with checklists and action cards, or consist of a loose collection of standing procedures coordinated through a group of people who are nominated to come together during a crisis to manage the event. Most will have some form of paper document, which will be known as the 'emergency plan', as confirmation of the arrangements. This chapter identifies the different types of emergency plans and their basic structure, and discusses the process approach to drafting, maintaining and amending such plans.

5.2 Types of emergency plans

Plans fall into three main categories: generic, site specific, and subject or function specific.

5.2.1 Generic plans

Generic plans are very broad in nature and seek to cover a range of possible risks, utilising many if not all of the facilities available from the organisation. These plans tend to provide the basic framework within which other, more specific emergency arrangements will be contained. They are often used as a policy document to drive the organisation's response and may not contain details of matters such as activation, resources, etc., their principal role being to outline the organisation's key role(s) and responsibilities.

5.2.2 Site-specific plans

Site-specific plans are those developed for specific locations, outlining a location's response to a clearly identified risk or series of risks. These plans are more clearly defined and would contain all the activities necessary to activate staff and resources, manage the situation and return the area to normality. Examples of these would be fire, chemical spill or physical damage, evacuation plans, and plans for loss of facilities such as power or water.

5.2.3 Subject- or function-specific plans

As the name implies, these types of plan are related to specific subject areas and functions, such as communications, a hostage situation, media management, or chemical, biological, radiological and nuclear (CBRN) incidents and mass casualty situations. Normally subject-/function-specific plans form part of a family of plans as specific arrangements within a generic plan, and they might be found as annexes within the major incident plan for a Trust.

5.3   Plan structure

This section provides a general overview of plan structure. More specific guidance on plan contents is contained both in the plan checklists in the annexes, which form part of the auditing process for Acute Trusts, PCTs and Ambulance Trusts, as well as in Criterion 3 of the Controls Assurance Standards for Emergency Planning in Chapter 6. The precise nature and style will depend on the type of Trust, its specific emergency planning needs and the in-house style of information dissemination. In general terms, an emergency plan would contain the following main sections, loosely grouped into three main headings:

- the generic introduction to the plan

- the emergency section

- the annexes.

5.3.1 The generic introduction to the plan

This section is very important in giving a clear overview as to what the plan is seeking to achieve. This may be laid out as a specific aim and range of objectives, or as a policy statement indicating what the plan seeks to accomplish. Information relating to how the plan is managed, who is responsible for updates, and how and when the plan is circulated, should also be included. This section may also contain a statement from the Chief Executive providing a clear statement of management involvement and endorsement, while underscoring the fact that the plan and the process behind its production are part of the requirement/service delivery of the Trust. The introductory section may also contain information on the range and extent of the identified hazards and associated risks in the area of responsibility for the Trust, including the anticipated effects on service delivery. This introductory section plays no part in the activation of the plan, so to avoid delay in using the plan in an emergency a number of Trusts include a clear statement to readers stating: 'In an emergency go straight to the section containing your action card.'

5.3.2 The emergency section

This section will contain the emergency activities needed to respond to and deal with the incident(s). A number of specific activities will fall under this general heading, such as:

- activation

- communications

- roles and responsibilities

- liaison and coordination arrangements, and

- recovery.

Activation

This section can also be seen as a subject-specific plan in its own right. This is normally presented in the form of a set of specific actions (sometimes with specific function- or role-based action cards and log sheets for recording activities). Alert may be scaled up through a number of levels such as Major Incident Standby and Major Incident Alert. This section would normally contain the internal mechanism for 'stand down'.

Communications

This is often presented as a separate section in many plans, mainly due to the critical nature of internal and external communications needs. It may contain details of specific message handling methods, and include logging, recording and data capture for legal and debriefing purposes.

Roles and responsibilities

The identification of who has overall responsibility within the Trust, and the specific roles of departments and individuals, should be set out in this section. This section may also contain the information needed to access additional resources. This is mostly achieved through the use of action cards and/or checklists to ensure a consistent approach. See Box 5.1 for an example of an action card.

Box 5.1 Example of an action card

ACTION CARD 27

Facilities Coordinator

- You will be advised by the hospital telephonist that a major incident has been declared. **Contact** one of the duty mangers who have agreed to act as the Public Relations Officer. **Contact** the Catering Manager, Sterile Services Manager, Hospital Security Officer and Car Park Manager.
- **Liaise** with Telecommunications Manager regarding provision of direct dialling facilities on phones required by certain key personnel.
- **Liaise** with Portering Services Manager or Senior Porter regarding the portering staff's response to a major incident as required in Action Card no. 33.
- **Liaise** with hospital telephonists to assess their ability to cope with the situation and provide management advice if needed.
- **Make** telephone available at Entrance 4 reception.
- **Liaise** with hospital coordination team to determine other support service requirement. Take action where necessary.
- **Liaise** with Hospital Security Officer regarding security of hospital areas and property that have been exposed to the general public outside normal working hours.
- **Stand down** will be declared by hospital coordination team when it is considered appropriate.
- Some support services will need to continue a 'special' service after 'stand down', i.e. telephones and catering. **Liaise with those concerned.**

Liaison and coordination arrangements

All inter-department, inter-health service organisation and external liaison should be indicated, including roles and responsibilities and contact details.

Recovery

This section, often overlooked, might include issues such as physical reconstruction (in the event of internal damage), replenishing stocks, taking stock of costs, payment for resources used, staff welfare and debrief and feedback arrangements. It may also include medium- to long-term public health monitoring of patient caseloads, e.g. following a chemical incident or environmental exposure where long-term effects need to be monitored.

5.3.3 Annexes

Internal plans, such as fire and evacuation arrangements, should be presented in this section, along with special arrangements for chemical, biological, radiological and nuclear (CBRN) incidents (see Chapter 10), media management (see Chapter 11) and mass casualty situations (see Chapter 10).

5.4   Plan process

To achieve a consistent approach to the development and maintenance of emergency plans, it is important to adopt an emergency planning process. Though many good emergency plan frameworks exist, it is important to ensure that plans are developed to suit the exact needs of the Trust for which they are intended. A process approach ensures a thorough investigation of the changing nature of the range of hazards and level of risk posed to the Trust, and ensures that the ever-changing nature of the organisation can adapt and react to the identified response needs. Following a systematic yet dynamic process ensures that the organisation more readily accepts and incorporates emergency planning into its management culture, thus reducing the negative perception that emergency planning is a 'bolt-on' operation and not part of the core activity of the Trust.

To achieve this there are a number of 'steps' to be taken, as follows:

- define the project
- develop and review the planning group
- analyse the potential problems
- determine mitigation strategies
- prepare the response requirement:
  - determine roles and responsibilities
  - analyse resources
- describe management structures
- develop sub-routines.

Each of these steps contains a number of specific activities that need to be covered. Further details of many of these activities are covered elsewhere in this handbook.

5.4.1 Defining the project

This is an important step in the process, one that will determine the aim, objectives and scope of an emergency plan while driving the tasks required for the project through the planning group (see below).

The requirement to plan

When addressing this issue, planners must be fully aware of the context in which they are being required to produce or amend an emergency plan. Is this the first plan of its type for the Trust? Are we being directed to develop the whole plan or part of a plan, or are we being asked to review or rewrite an existing plan? What is the relationship of this plan with others within and external to the Trust? Will our activities impinge on others already making or completing plans that may overlap with our emergency plan? Careful consideration must therefore be given to the legislation and guidance relating to the type and content of the plan (see Chapter 2).

The scope of the plan

What geographic or organisational area will the plan cover? Does this relate to one or more sites or to a geographical boundary such as a county, Strategic Health Authority or PCT boundary? Some of these boundaries are both geographical and organisational, and are not coterminous. Therefore, how will this effect your plan process and the content of the plan?

Will all or part of the plan be time limited? Will parts of the plan be time specific, such as winter pressures or one-off carnivals or sporting occasions? If so, the process lead-in time needs to reflect this, i.e. the plan review time frames must be carefully considered to ensure any revisions or updates for the plan are not rushed at the last minute before the event.

5.4.2 Developing and reviewing the planning group

Any emergency planning group must be relevant to the needs of the project. All participants should be competent and enthusiastic, and have the authority to commit the organisation or unit they represent. Emergency planning groups can easily be bogged down if group members are not aware of the task or competent to provide information regarding their group's/organisation's input without continuous reference to a higher authority, or when they are not committed to their role. The size of any group may from time to time fluctuate with the needs of the project. To facilitate the group, all decisions should be recorded and circulated to members. The style and font size, etc. should be decided on early in the meetings to reduce time delays and frustrations during the drafting and editing stages of the plan's production.

5.4.3 Analysing potential problems

All forms of threats to a Trust, and all forms of hazard relating to a Trust's service delivery, must be assessed through a formal 'hazard analysis'. This should take into account the worst-case scenario and include all possible combinations. Following the hazard analysis a 'risk assessment' should be carried out to determine the level of risk. This is normally described simply as *high, medium* or *low*. In doing so, the *frequency* and *severity* should be taken into account, along with people's perception of the risk (see Chapter 4).

5.4.4 Determining mitigation strategies

This element can be better described as 'risk reduction methods'. Many emergency planners do not see this activity as part of their remit; however, during the emergency planning process, it is essential that you are aware of the possibility of identifying and reducing risk within the Trust, particularly for threats from within the organisation/buildings you are planning for. This can take the form of simple strategies to reduce fire risks in conjunction with your health and safety team, or reducing or separating high-risk storage through negotiations with the responsible managers. In addition, when consulting with outside agencies, you should be aware of the need to reduce risk wherever possible, and be prepared to offer guidance to outside agencies on their risk reduction role. Risk reduction (see Chapter 4) measures that can be implemented or recommended include:

- separation of high-risk storage
- spatial planning changes (advice to outside agencies)
- design changes
- safety training
- security.

5.4.5 Preparing the response requirement

Determining roles and responsibilities

Roles and responsibilities must be defined and described to ensure that each organisation, Trust and department/unit knows exactly what is expected of it, and to ensure that people are aware of the general roles of all relevant organisations within the scope of the plan. The definition of roles and responsibilities may also assist in defining jobs outside the normal activity of Trust staff, eliminating obvious gaps, clarifying resource needs, ensuring durability and compatibility, and avoiding 'double counting'. In relation to the overall emergency, this activity will determine who is the primary (or lead) agency for given types of emergency, and who are the secondary (or support) agencies.

Analysing resources

Clarifying roles and responsibilities will lead to analysing resources. It is important to determine needs, identify sources and prepare the access. This activity will ensure that 'just in time' delivery systems, which operate during normal working practices, can cope with the increased demand that will be placed on them in an emergency. Critical thinking will need to be applied to ensure that all possible resources can be accessed at all times of the day and night, and that replenishment systems are durable even at weekends and on bank holidays. Where human and/or physical resources are needed at the scene, adequate fallback arrangements should be considered to ensure that the deployment of these resources does not leave a crucial activity without cover within the Trust.

Roles and responsibilities are often extended into action cards for use by staff in the event of an emergency – these should be brief but thorough. Consideration needs to be given to the nature of the roles and the extent to which individuals will be working outside of their normal activity. The action card should act as an aide-memoire to those simply performing their own specialism within the context of an emergency, whereas individuals performing general roles outside of their specialism should be given specific instructions along with short, concise guidance notes. All staff likely to use action cards *must* be given a full briefing on their role within an emergency plan, and be provided with an opportunity to practise that role on a regular basis.

5.4.6 Describing management structures

The management structure concerns the authority and reporting relationships within and between departments/units and different organisations. There needs to be a clear and shared understanding of internal and external relationships in order for organisations to minimise confusion during emergencies. Moreover, there needs to be agreement on the management structure among each and every department/unit and organisation involved in the plan. There are also a number of concepts commonly used for management structures. The terms 'command', 'control' and 'coordination' are often used to describe how incidents and crises are managed:

- 'Command' is the direction of the members and resources of an organisation in the performance of its role and tasks. Command relates to organisations and operates vertically within the organisation.

- 'Control' is the overall direction of emergency activities. Authority for control is established in legislation or in a plan and carries with it the responsibility for tasking and coordinating other organisations in accordance with the needs of the situation. Therefore control relates to situations and operates horizontally.

- 'Coordination' is the harmonious integration of the expertise of all the agencies involved, with the object of effectively and efficiently bringing the incident to a successful conclusion.

Management structures are often presented as a structure diagram showing the command features within departments and units of an organisation, and the control features between organisations working together towards a common goal. Specific features may include:

- call-out arrangements
- coordination arrangements
- command and control structures
- channels of communication
- multi-agency/cross-border arrangements.

5.4.7 Development of sub-routines

The final element in the process to produce an emergency plan is the generation of sub-routines or subject-/function-specific plans in support of the main plan. Subject- or function-specific plans will in their own right also need to be developed using the same process as for the emergency plan within which they sit. This process should (because of the work previously undertaken) be truncated, but should still be carried out in a similar manner to ensure completeness. Care should be taken with these sub-plans to ensure compatibility between them and with the main (generic) plan. Special attention should be given to the issue of double-earmarking of staff and equipment, and to ensuring that the delivery of any of the support mechanisms to the main plan is timely. Typical examples are as follows:

- emergency control rooms
- information gathering and data storage
- evacuation plans
- public warning and alerting systems
- resource procurement
- press and public relations arrangements
- welfare plans for survivors and staff
- communications plans
- business continuity
- recovery plans.

The case study described in Box 5.2 provides an example of how an Acute Trust identified and carried out a full review of its major incident plan.

Box 5.2 St Bartholomew's and the Royal London Trust: a Trust perspective of reviewing emergency planning

Following the terrorist attack in New York on 11 September 2001, St Bartholomew's and the Royal London (BLT), like most NHS Trusts, undertook a thorough review of its level of preparedness to respond to an event of such magnitude. The Trust has a wealth of experience in responding to most of the major incidents that have occurred in London over the past twenty years, but on reviewing the plan it was clear that adjustments would be needed in order to respond to a catastrophic event.

The Chief Nurse was designated by the Chief Executive as the lead director with responsibility for emergency planning, and convened an executive-level planning team. In addition to executive leadership, a project manager was appointed (who had a strong clinical nursing background) to work full time on secondment to the Emergency Planning Liaison Officer (EPLO) and executive lead, to ensure the Major Incident Planning Group's action plans were managed in a systematic and effective way.

The Major Incident Planning Group has met monthly since October 2001. Each clinical director and general manager has been charged to ensure local major incident plans are developed within each speciality and submitted for approval to the Major Incident Planning Group. The revised major incident plan was produced in a clear format, and included the most up-to-date guidance. The plan itself was reviewed by the Regional Health Emergency Planning Adviser (RHEPA).

Once the hospital plan was completed, a detailed work programme was put in place to ensure all clinical directorates, wards and departments had robust major incident local plans in place. These were systematically reviewed by the Major Incident Planning Group to ensure consistency in terms of style and fit within the overall organisation for the Trust's response.

Within the major incident plan itself, there is provision for 'special incidents'. The Major Incident Planning Group believed this was essential to avoid overreaction while ensuring systematic management of events which would fall under the following headings: 'the rising tide', 'cloud on the horizon', 'headline news', and some internal incidents. In addition to the immediate response from clinical teams and departments, two areas became very clear to the planning group, areas which needed careful attention and thoughtful construction. The first was to ensure that robust responses from the facilities directorate were in place; the second was the confirmation of location(s) and arrangements for the formation of the hospital control team.

The designation of the facilities directorate within a major incident is essential to ensure that support services are immediately available to facilitate smooth execution of the major incident plan. Of particular importance was well-briefed facilities staff in the security, portering and catering departments. Clear signposting, crowd control and security are fundamental to the underpinning of an effective major incident response.

In terms of the hospital control team, it became clear that a generic action card was required for members. The hospital control team is comprised of medical, nursing, management and facilities presence. In the first instance, the hospital control team consists of the Nurse-in-Charge of the emergency department, the duty A&E Consultant and the Site Manager. Over a period of time, appropriate on-call staff replace the on-site staff with senior members of staff representing the Chief Executive, Medical Director and Chief Nurse. The hospital control team has a number of control room locations, allowing operational resilience should the incident become protracted or necessitate building closure.

A comprehensive and systematic training programme was developed for all staff, including abbreviated briefing documents for new starters and the production of a new video, which would be used for training purposes across the Trust. Once the major incident plan had been completed, a large tabletop exercise was held, at which every directorate was present and the whole plan exercised in its constituent parts. Amendments were made to the plan and further exercises were carried out within directorates, in order for detailed amendments to be made to local plans. In addition to the local exercises, the Trust participated in exercises run by the PCT and the Strategic Health Authority.

The major incident plan itself is posted on a major incident website as part of the Trust's intranet. All local plans are also on the website, with hyperlinks to appropriate national websites, in particular the Health Protection Agency and other government resources.

Jonathan E. Asbridge
Chief Nurse of St Bartholomew's and the Royal London

5.5 Relationship with business continuity planning

Whilst the emergency plan deals with the organisation of the necessary response to (normally) rapid-onset emergencies or disaster, business continuity planning deals with the continuity of service within an organisation during times of crisis, be it a crisis created by an emergency such as failure of power or water supply, or service disruption such as loss of a supplier. All Trusts should consider business continuity management as a strategic management issue.

It is also necessary to consider continuity of service during the implementation of a major incident plan. All parts of the Trust can be affected by the knock-on effect of the range of activities needed to respond to the major incident. The hospital management team must take this into account when dealing with the strategic issues emanating from the emergency response. It is also essential to consider how other parts of the service, those not directly involved in the response to the emergency, are properly maintained as resources and staff from core services are redirected to the emergency response. Careful consideration should therefore be given as to how the major incident plan dovetails with business continuity management within the Trust. It is essential that these two disciplines are seen as being mutually supportive, *not* mutually exclusive.

5.6 Summary

This chapter provided an overview of the different types of emergency plans, their basic structure and content. Most importantly, the chapter has explored the process needed to encompass the many facets of emergency planning into a cohesive set of planning arrangements, which will promote an integrated and coordinated response to a major incident.

6 Plan Evaluation and Audit

Sarah Norman

6.1 Introduction

Plans need to be viewed as living documents, evolving, changing and adapting continuously. 'This cycle of learning needs to be repeated regularly whether or not a major incident has occurred' (Department of Health 1998). The cycle of learning is represented in Figure 6.1.

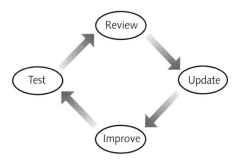

Figure 6.1 Cycle of learning (adapted from Department of Health 1998)

The Department of Health requires that major incident plans are reviewed on an annual basis, and more frequently when there have been changes to organisations or personnel that could affect the response to a major incident (Department of Health 1998).

The reviewing and auditing of plans, arrangements or emergency preparedness should be viewed as an opportunity to identify best practice, which can then be shared with other colleagues and Trusts.

It is envisaged that a national audit tool will be developed, which may encompass and build on some or all of the following methods. The current methods of reviewing plans and auditing preparedness include:

- self-assessment checklists for plans
- the 8Cs of preparedness
- Controls Assurance Standards for Emergency Planning.

6.2 Self-assessment checklist of plans

A number of self-assessment checklists have been developed by the Regional Health Emergency Planning Advisers (RHEPAs) to allow Trusts to assess their plans and arrangements against set criteria.[1] The three types of self-assessment checklist are designed for:

- Acute Trusts
- Primary Care Trusts (can also be used for Non-Acute Trusts)
- Ambulance Trusts.

The checklists are available on the Department of Health website (www.dh.gov.uk) and can also be found in the annexes of this handbook.

The assessment tools incorporate all of the essential elements that should be included in a PCT, Ambulance Trust and Acute Trust major incident plan. Each checklist is a combination of Department of Health national guidance and good practice; they reflect current thinking and National Health Service (NHS) structures, and offer a framework for trust emergency planning. The tools were developed by the RHEPAs and designed to support Trust emergency planning, and can be used in several ways.

For individual Trust's to self-assess their emergency plans in order to identify any gaps, areas of weakness, strength and training needs of the organisation.

It is intended that when a Trust has used this tool for self assessment an action plan is drawn up to address areas of weakness, to fill any planning gaps, and to establish a corporate training programme and, most importantly, who is going to take forward any work (within what timescales) to ensure progress is made. Any action plan should be endorsed by the Trust Executive Board to engender corporate ownership and identification of appropriate funding for implementation of the action plan.

The tool also allows external assessors (usually RHEPAs) to make a determination of the Trust's level of emergency preparedness.

In so doing it allows the RHEPA to work with the Trust on identified problem areas and offer appropriate training and support. It also allows the RHEPA an opportunity to consider where there is scope for additional joint working at a local or regional level.

The assessment tools have been endorsed by the Department of Health and should be used in conjunction with the Controls Assurance Standards for Emergency Planning for Trusts. They should act as an aide-memoire to facilitate robust health emergency planning within your organisation, enhance organisational resilience and build local public confidence in the integrity of an individual PCT's level of preparedness.

6.3 The 8Cs of preparedness

The National Audit Office (NAO)(2002) report, *Facing the Challenge: NHS Emergency Planning in England*, whilst showing that progress is being made, also raised some significant concerns. The NHS needed to be able to demonstrate that it responded constructively to the recommendations in the report. As such, the Director of Operations for the Department of Health set out 'How to assess preparedness?' by developing the '8Cs of preparedness' from Annex F of the NAO report. The '8Cs' approach recognises that the physical 'plan' is a key component of preparedness, but also that emergency preparedness needs to be viewed holistically to include 'readiness, including ownership and understanding within the Trust, training and the availability of the right equipment and procedures' (Doran 2003). The 8Cs are summarised as follows:

> **Clarity** – are roles and responsibilities within and between organisations clear and defined? Who is in charge?
>
> **Coherence** – are the respective functions of all relevant players known and understood by each of them? Do they fit together?

Contingencies – are different operational possibilities and threats accounted for? Are the plans (and the underpinning arrangements) flexible without being vague?

Collaboration – a basic principle is that of mutual aid and support with neighbouring and partner organisations; this must be spelled out in specific terms as well as principles.

Credibility – plans and processes, to be credible, must have been put to the test within a valid time period.

Capability – are the right skills and expertise available to meet the likely scale of threat? The training and testing of staff, equipment and procedures must be demonstrated to be up to date against an appropriate schedule.

Communications – do the plans make plain how communicating with staff, patients and the public will be achieved effectively?

Commitment – there must be evidence of commitment to the plan and supporting arrangements, and their up-dating, by all members of the board and, in PCTs or in hospital trusts, the Hospital Medical Committee or its equivalent (Doran 2003).

The 8Cs continue to be useful indicators of preparedness, and Trusts may be asked in the future annually to assess their level of preparedness against this framework. Historically, the RHEPA was responsible for reviewing plans with individual Trusts; however, following the development of the 8Cs of preparedness, each Strategic Health Authority was expected to review the plans and arrangements in every one of their Trusts and to confirm that these were satisfactory. The capacity and expertise to undertake such a role was not available in many Strategic Health Authorities and will need to be developed with the RHEPAs, as it may form part of the performance management role of Strategic Health Authorities.

6.4 Controls Assurance Standards for Emergency Planning

The Controls Assurance Standards (www.hcsu.org.uk), developed by Keele University, form part of the auditing process required of all NHS organisations (Department of Health 2002a) (also stated in the Department of Health (2004) document, *Handling Major Incidents: An Operational Doctrine*).[2] The Controls Assurance Standard for Emergency Planning states:

> The organisation has planned and prepared an organised and practised response to all major incidents and emergency situations which affect the provision of normal services. The purpose of planning for emergencies in the NHS is to ensure preparedness for an effective response to any major incident or emergency and to ensure that the organisation fully recovers to normal services as quickly as possible. The standard applies to the ability of the organisation to:
>
> - respond to incidents which are outside their normal experience and which are of such a scale that special arrangements are necessary
>
> - contribute effectively to the combined response of all the emergency services and other agencies.

All NHS organisations should already have detailed major incident plans, which are tested and reviewed at least on an annual basis. The standard mirrors the key requirements of NHS emergency planning guidance.

The overall aim of major incident planning is to achieve an effective response to an incident regardless of its cause. Plans should be sufficiently flexible to deal with a range of situations that are likely to increase in significance, duration and complexity, and which may affect more than one health region, commissioning authority, provider or service.

The planning process should ensure that the organisation has:

- assessed the hazards and risks
- a wide, whole population approach to situations which may affect their own and neighbouring health and social care economies, including mass casualty incidents
- identified internal and external dependencies
- collaborated within the health service and with other associated organisations
- communications strategies and procedures in place to deal with any incident within the scope of major incident and service continuity planning
- effective training and testing programmes in place
- effective review, refinement and performance monitoring procedures in place
- taken children's, ethnic, religious and cultural needs into account
- version and distribution control of all plans.

Box 6.1 Auditing obligations in the Operational Doctrine

The Doctrine (Department of Health 2004) states:

- **All NHS bodies already have an obligation under the Controls Assurance process to assess their compliance with emergency planning requirements. This is now re-stated in terms of this doctrine.**
- All NHS bodies must now ensure that they review, improve and have a programme for regularly testing their plans and that those are reported at Board level. Annual reports for 2003/4 must include a Controls Assurance statement signed by Chief Executives certifying that their organisation has major incident plans in place which are fully compliant with this doctrine and accompanying NHS guidance on major incident preparedness and planning.

The Controls Assurance Standard for Emergency Planning comprises of 12 criteria, as described below.

CRITERION 1

Board level responsibility for emergency planning is clearly defined and there are clear lines of accountability throughout the organisation, leading to the board.

Guidance

The key requirements are that the organisation should demonstrate that:

- the Chief Executive accepts overall responsibility for major incident planning and has appointed and given authority to a senior and experienced manager or clinician to lead the planning team

- key roles and responsibilities are defined, including clarity on who will lead on different aspects of the response
- key staff understand and are competent to fulfil their roles
- emergency response arrangements are integrated into the organisation's everyday working structure and processes
- annual business plans should address individual and group training requirements to maintain an effective major incident response.

Examples of verification

- Evidence of the board meeting(s) at which a report on emergency planning was received
- Key roles and responsibilities are written within emergency planning documents and service agreements
- Evidence of an emergency planning group which meets regularly
- Emergency planning responsibilities, including the need to train, included in job descriptions.

CRITERION 2

There is a major incident plan for the organisation.

Guidance

The organisation should demonstrate that there is a written plan in place to respond to both internal and external emergency situations. The key requirements are:

- The plan is in accordance with the national emergency planning guidance
- The plan should be structured to achieve an overall emergency response regardless of the underlying cause.

The plan should include:

- The criteria to be used to define a major incident or emergency situation
- Assessment of local hazards and risks
- Potential detrimental effects on normal service provision
- The identification of who has overall responsibility at the time that the major incident or emergency is declared
- Effective alerting arrangements
- A control and coordination mechanism and procedures
- Robust and diverse means of communication
- Arrangements for collaboration within the NHS and with others
- The provision of health care and welfare in the exceptional circumstances that may prevail after a major incident
- Liaison and coordination arrangements
- The provision of regular and accurate information to the public and the media.

Examples of verification

- Evidence of a current plan for the organisation, which incorporates all of the above aspects.

CRITERION 3

All feasible/realistic types of emergency situations are addressed in the service continuity plan(s).

Guidance

Major incidents and emergencies cross many departments, organisations, providers and boundaries, with incidents arising directly and indirectly from many situations. Failures may be serial, single or multiple, concurrent, organisational, regional or national. Risk and impact analysis can be used to identify how failures will affect the organisation from any of these situations.

The failures may impact directly onto the plan itself through failure of communication systems, electricity or transport, for example. Dependency modelling can usefully be used to identify the dynamic links and priorities of the dependencies and thus help eliminate gaps that failures may create. Plans should include risks to both operational and technical failures. The process contained in the risk management standard will guide the above.

Examples of verification

- Evidence of current supporting documentation for the plan, detailing the process of risk and hazard identification, methods of risk reduction, scenarios of possible failures, modes of failure and impact for the organisation, taking account of the above aspects
- Business continuity document.

CRITERION 4

All internal and external stakeholders in the major incident plan are consulted and collaborated with concerning their roles and responsibilities.

Guidance

Very infrequently do emergency situations arise which affect health-care organisations in isolation. Thus, in the planning process for major incidents, it is critical to consider and involve all potential internal and external stakeholders. There should be:

- integration with external agencies
- liaison with other partner NHS agencies
- encouragement to staff to contribute to planning and preparation for a major incident.

Examples of verification

- Evidence of NHS representation on multi-agency planning groups
- A nominated representative within all relevant NHS organisations
- Evidence of an internal emergency planning group with representatives from all relevant departments.

CRITERION 5

Emergency preparedness is validated through the exercising and testing of emergency plans.

Guidance

All emergency plans should be tested, in exercises, to ensure their effectiveness. The following are key requirements:

- The regular in-house testing of major incident plans
- Live exercises every three years (Ambulance Service annually)
- Multi-agency testing and exercising of plans
- Communications exercises every six months (Ambulance Service monthly)
- There is comprehensive debriefing of exercises.

Examples of verification

- Evidence that exercises have been carried out
- All opportunities have been taken for multi-agency involvement in exercises
- Evidence of switchboard and other staff training in the cascade of alerting messages
- Production of debriefing reports.

CRITERION 6

The major incident plan is regularly reviewed.

Guidance

The major incident plan should be fully reviewed on an annual basis or more frequently where service changes or improvement evidence from the activation of the plan indicates. This will ensure that the arrangements are still valid and that training for incidents and emergencies is still appropriate, and that there is full commitment to the plan.

The review process should address and validate all elements and organisations that form part of the plan. This should include:

- Evidence of an annual independent audit of the major incident plan by the Health Emergency Planning Adviser (HEPA) or other suitably qualified person
- Evidence of review and amendment of the major incident plan.

Examples of verification

- Evidence of an annual independent audit of the major incident plan
- Evidence of review and amendment of the major incident plan.

CRITERION 7

The organisation provides funding and resources to ensure that emergency planning responsibilities are met and that it is able to respond effectively to a major incident.

Guidance

All capital and revenue costs relating to emergency planning should be clearly identified and included within the business planning and budgetary arrangements for

NHS organisations. NHS organisations should ensure that funds have been allocated to the following key areas:

- Staffing
- Preparation and production of plans and action cards
- Staff training and participation in exercises
- Communications equipment
- Appropriate specialist facilities
- Appropriate specialist personal protective clothing and equipment.

Examples of verification

- The availability of plans and action cards
- The availability and serviceability of facilities, equipment and stores
- Evidence of budgetary allocation.

CRITERION 8

The organisation has access to up-to-date guidance relating to emergency planning.

Guidance

Access to relevant guidance is essential. As a minimum, those involved in emergency planning should have access to the key references, in particular:

- HSC 1998/197
- Department of Health (1998), *Planning for Major Incidents: The NHS Guidance* (London: HMSO)
- Cabinet Office (2003), *Dealing with Disaster* (3rd edn)(London: Brodie Publishing Ltd)
- Home Office (1998), *The Exercise Planner's Guide: A Guide to Testing Emergency Arrangements* (London: HMSO)
- Department of Health (2000), *Deliberate Release of Biological and Chemical Agents: Guidance to Help Plan the Health Service's Response* (London: Department of Health)
- The Department of Health COIN database (www.dh.gov.uk)
- The Health Care Standards Unit website (www.hcsu.org.uk)
- The Emergency Planning College at Easingwold website (www.ukresilience.info/college/index.htm)
- The Department of Health Emergency Planning Co-ordination Unit website (www.dh.gov.uk/epcu/index.htm).

Examples of verification

- Demonstration of internet access and/or NHS net
- Availability of key references.

CRITERION 9

All staff receive emergency preparedness training that is commensurate with their role in the major incident plan.

Guidance

Almost all staff could be involved in responding to a major incident. All staff should, therefore, have appropriate knowledge of the major incident plan commensurate with their roles and responsibilities. For those who are likely to have a key role in the response there must be regular training. The following are key requirements:

- Annual business plan to address individual and group training

- Development of a training programme

- Regular in-house training for staff who have a specific role in a major incident response

- Ensure that staff are familiar with the use of specialist facilities and equipment

- Mobile Medical Teams and Medical Incident Officers are trained as appropriate.

Examples of verification

- Evidence that key staff have attended external multi-agency and NHS training courses

- Personal training records

- Induction training records.

CRITERION 10

Key indicators capable of showing improvements in emergency preparedness and/or providing early warning of risk are used at all levels of the organisation, including the board, and the efficacy and usefulness of the indicators is reviewed regularly.

Guidance

The organisation should develop indicators, which demonstrate the risk associated with the resilience of the system in place for emergency preparedness. One indicator is degree of compliance with this standard. Ideally the indicators should be designed to demonstrate improvement in the performance of the system over time. The number of indicators devised should be sufficient to monitor the system. It is not necessarily the case that all the indicators will be used by the board. The board should select those which are useful for ensuring that the internal controls are working satisfactorily and that the system in place is meeting its objectives.

The Department of Health will review the actual indicators used by organisations to identify best practice in indicator use. This will inform the development of a set of national indicators for 'high-level' benchmarking and monitoring purposes.

Examples of verification

- Indicators

- Evidence of usage at all levels.

CRITERION 11

The system in place for emergency planning and preparedness is monitored and reviewed by management and the board in order to make improvements to the system.

Guidance

It is the responsibility of the Chief Executive and the board to monitor and review all aspects of the system for emergency planning, including:

- accountability arrangements
- processes, including risk management arrangements
- capability
- outcomes
- internal audit findings.

An emergency planning committee or group may exist to carry out detailed reviews. The risk management committee will play a significant role in monitoring and reviewing all aspects of the system as a basis for establishing significant information that should be presented to and dealt with by the board. The Audit Committee should review internal audit findings.

Examples of verification

- Internal audit report(s)
- Audit Committee minutes
- Emergency planning committee/group minutes
- Risk management committee minutes.

CRITERION 12

The board seeks independent assurance that an appropriate and effective system of managing emergency planning is in place and that the necessary level of controls and monitoring is being implemented.

Guidance

Management should consider the range of independent internal and external assurance available, and avoid duplication and omission. The adequacy of the independent assurance will depend upon the scope and depth of the work performed, bearing in mind its timeliness and the competency of the staff performing it. The level of reliance that can be placed upon such assurances should consider, among other things, the professional standing of the assurers, their level of independence, and whether they could reasonably expect to provide an objective opinion. It is important that any review that takes place results in a report, recommendations for action where necessary, and the retention of sufficient evidence to enable other potential reviewers to rely upon the work already undertaken. The reports should be made to the appropriate sub-committee of the board.

Management arrangements will include an internal audit function, as well as other quality control and assurance functions such as clinical audit. The internal audit function is required to give an opinion to the board on the adequacy and effectiveness of the overall system of internal control. In doing so, they will seek to work with, and rely on the work of, other review bodies as far as is practical. The NHS is given external assurance by such bodies as:

- external auditors, as appointed by the Audit Commission
- Healthcare Commission (previously known as the Commission for Health Improvement).

More specific assurance for this standard may be gained from visits by:

- Health and Safety Executive
- Health Emergency Planning Adviser.

Examples of verification
- Schedule of planned reviews
- Copy of reports
- Committee minutes.

6.5 Summary

The Department of Health requires major incident plans to be reviewed on an annual basis, and more frequently when there have been changes to organisations or personnel that could affect the response to a major incident (Department of Health 1998). Given this requirement, this chapter has provided an overview of the three types of auditing methods used in the NHS. It is envisaged that a national audit tool, when developed, will build on these methods.

6.6 Notes

1. Section 6.2 is reproduced from Wheatley (2003), with the kind permission of the author.

2. The information about Controls Assurance Standards for Emergency Planning in section 6.4, including the 12 criteria, has been reproduced with the kind permission of Crown Copyright 2002.

7

Planning Exercises and Training

Sarah Norman

7.1 Introduction

Following the development of your major incident plan, or following a major incident, a programme of exercising and training should be planned to ensure your staff are suitably prepared and your plan is appropriately tested. 'After any exercise, the plan should be reviewed and amended from lessons learned before the process starts again' (Home Office 1998). The process of training and exercising is summarised in Figure 7.1. This chapter outlines some of the key elements about planning exercises and training.

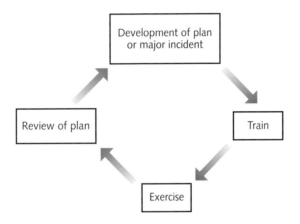

Figure 7.1 Process of training and exercising (Department of Health 1998)

7.2 Training

Training involves:[1]

- ensuring that staff have the right skills and knowledge to undertake the roles expected of them in a major incident
- familiarising all staff, particularly new staff, with special equipment or systems
- testing the major incident plan by appropriate exercises
- assessing plans and training needs as part of an ongoing cycle of quality improvement.

It is essential to assess the skills expected of staff who plan for or respond to a major incident, and whether staff in post have those skills. You will need a carefully planned and delivered major incident training programme so that staff:

- understand their roles and the roles of others and how these relate to each other
- understand their major incident plan's systems and procedures

- know how accommodation should be used
- know where equipment is kept and how to use it
- make necessary preparations
- perform to an agreed standard
- learn from experience.

Box 7.1 Training ideas

Less formal training can be undertaken to promote emergency planning as part of day-to-day work practices. For example:

- organise guest presentations on relevant topics at regular staff meetings, away days or lunchtimes
- organise practical hands-on training, e.g. arrange for your Ambulance Trust to demonstrate the pods and allow staff to have a 'play' with the equipment
- organise experiential media training for those within your Trust who are likely be in contact with the media during a major incident.

Training involves a significant investment in time and other resources. Your organisation will fully realise the benefits from this investment – people knowing what to do and how to do it – when training is planned and managed efficiently and effectively. If training is poorly targeted or badly executed, your investment will be of less value. Remember to document all who have been trained and all refreshers or updates. It may be sensible to keep copies of any training certification for future reference.

Developing the training programme

Consider the following when you are developing your major incident training programme.

- **Identify training needs**
  Who needs to be trained and what do they need to be trained to do? New staff must have their part in a major incident plan explained as part of their induction. Have organisational changes created a training need? How have people performed in exercises, major incidents or other crises?

- **Prioritise training needs**
  Given finite resources, what are your priorities?

- **Identify methods of training**
  There is a wide variety of training methods. Needs will vary according to roles, individual choice and personal circumstances. Training must be provided to suit individual requirements so far as possible. Consider:
  - selected reading: your organisation's major incident plan must come first
  - learning on the job
  - instructional videos and CD-ROMs
  - in-house group training sessions
  - locally arranged training with sector/county or Regional Health Emergency Planning Adviser (RHEPA)

- external courses, e.g. Civil Contingencies Secretariat (CCS), Emergency Planning College in Easingwold
- use of modular training to meet specific needs.
- **Get feedback**
Ask those who have been trained what worked well and what was of limited value.

Major incident plans must be reviewed annually or more frequently when service changes have an impact on the response. As part of such a review, Trusts should consider the training needs of staff.

7.3 Exercises

The choice and timing of exercises is important. Exercises should be organised in an appropriate and cost-effective way to ensure the aims and objectives are achieved. 'It is important to validate your major incident plan and the competencies of staff by appropriate exercises at regular intervals as part of your organisation's quality assurance and improvement programme' (Department of Health 1998). A well-run exercise:

- provides an important management tool for informing and motivating staff and building the confidence of those who may be asked to respond in a crisis
- brings together those likely to be involved in the response and allows them and their organisation to examine their performance under controlled conditions
- provides an assessment of the impact of an incident on the organisation and its ability to continue to provide its full range of essential health services
- identifies strengths and weaknesses of organisational systems
- identifies training needs of individuals
- tests whether lessons identified from previous exercises have been embedded into revised arrangements
- demonstrates commitment to quality to local stakeholders and external inquirers (adapted from Department of Health 1998).

In the Department of Health publication (1998) *Planning for Major Incidents*, the recommendation is for Trusts to undertake the following:

- a communications exercise every six months (or every month for Ambulance Trusts)
- a tabletop exercise every year
- a live exercise every three years (or every year for Ambulance Trusts).

7.3.1 Communications exercise

The aim of a communications exercise is (1) to exercise the call-out arrangements for major incident activation *within* the Trust, thereby improving the preparedness and capability of the Trust's response, or (2) to test the communications between Trusts and external agencies. Some Trusts may also set up their control room during a communications exercise, to test phone/fax lines and other aspects of setting up the room. The objectives may include:

- exercising the switchboard procedures for major incident alert
- testing the accuracy of the telephone/pager directory

- exercising the use of the major incident communications equipment and testing/checking its serviceability

- exercising the initial response of key post holders

- generating a 'snap-shot' of post holders' availability and estimated response times.

A communications exercise must *not* involve:

- the activation of the Trust's emergency management plan

- the cancellation or disruption of any Trust services

- the removal of staff from their posts if patient care is likely to be affected.

Box 7.2 When to facilitate a communications exercise

Consider running a communications exercise at different times of the day to see whether the response is the same. For example, your Trust could experiment using some of the following times:

- 7 a.m. or 11 a.m., or 6 p.m. or 3 a.m.
- during the weekend or on a bank holiday.

Key aspects of a communications exercise:

- Directing staff from the Trust should be identified in advance.

- The exercise begins when the Trust's switchboard is first notified by the local Ambulance Trust, Regional Health Emergency Planning Adviser (RHEPA) or other appropriate person. All exercise messages must begin and end with the word 'EXERCISE'. Directing staff must intervene if this is not the case.

- The exercise should continue until all those members of staff who have been paged/called have contacted the switchboard to provide the estimated time it would take for them to be in post from their current location.

- A 'hot' debrief (refer to Chapter 12 for further information on debriefing) for the switchboard staff must occur. The exercise log, 'hot' debrief notes and directing staff notes should be used to compile a written report into the exercise, which includes a section on 'lessons identified'.

- Any lessons identified from the communications exercise should be actioned and attached to any report. Copies of the report should be sent to the Trust's Chief Executive, Strategic Health Authority, sector/county EPLO (where in post) and RHEPA.

7.3.2 Tabletop exercise

The Home Office (1998) suggests tabletop exercises are a very cost-effective and efficient method of testing plans, procedures and people. They are difficult to run with large numbers, but those players who are involved are provided with an excellent opportunity to interact with and understand the roles and responsibilities of the other agencies or players taking part. They can engage players imaginatively and generate high levels of realism. Participants will get to know realistic key procedures along with the people with whom they may be working in an emergency. Those who have exercised together and know each other will provide a much more effective response than those who come together for the first time when a disaster occurs. An element of media awareness can be introduced under controlled conditions, such as the preparation of press releases at the tactical level, or the use of trainee journalists, under the direction of their tutors, to play news-hungry reporters (Home Office 1998).

The objectives of a tabletop exercise may include:

- exercising the plan using a realistic scenario
- testing the accuracy of procedures, instructions or actions listed within the plan
- testing action cards for accuracy, appropriateness and clarity
- providing an opportunity for participants to get to know each other before a major incident occurs.

Box 7.3 Quick quiz

An exercise does not need to be an elaborately planned event. Small activities within the Trust, in between larger exercises, are extremely valuable for keeping emergency planning at the forefront of people's minds. Allow a little extra time in meetings or away-days, and throw in a quick-fire scenario. For example:

- What would happen within the Trust if you received a bomb threat now? What is the process for responding to such an incident within the Trust?
- How many staff do you have trained in personal protective equipment (PPE) on each shift? How long would it take to set up the area for decontamination if a no-notice incident occurred now?
- How would you clean your Trust if it was contaminated by self-presenting casualties? Consider contractors, staff involvement, welfare of staff and patients, etc.
- Consider how you could create extra capacity within your Trust if a major incident occurred involving large numbers of casualties. How could you access additional resources quickly?
- What are your considerations if, while responding to a major incident, you also have a power failure within the Trust? How will this affect your ability to respond to the major incident?

Key aspects of a tabletop exercise:

- Directing staff and umpires from the Trust should be identified in advance.
- A realistic time frame for completing the exercise should be established.
- There should be a realistic time frame for groups attending the exercise to discuss the scenario and insert questions.
- Providing opportunities for discussion and debate about issues arising.
- Ensuring comments, suggestions and discussions are logged.
- A 'hot' debrief (refer to Chapter 12 of this handbook for further information on debriefing) of participants must occur to ensure that any key issues, which urgently need to be resolved, can be raised. The exercise log, 'hot' debrief notes and directing staff notes should be used to compile a written report into the exercise, which includes a section on 'lessons identified'.

- Any lessons identified from the tabletop exercise should be actioned and attached to any report. Copies of the report should be made available to the Trust's Chief Executive, Strategic Health Authority, sector/county EPLO (where in post) and RHEPA.

Types of tabletop exercises:[2]

- **Time lapse exercise**

  It requires a decision to be made at an early stage as to whether the exercise will flow in real time or consist of 'snapshots' of time, i.e. a series of descriptions of how the scenario has progressed over time. For example, participants may spend a relatively short time considering the immediate actions to be taken, before moving to a scenario 'x hours into the incident' so that recovery issues can feature. Also consider whether exercise time will be stopped at any point during the exercise to allow for review or consideration of variables, e.g. weather, time of day or year.

- **Controlled play**

  In controlled exercises, the scenario and all events or incidents are pre-scripted. The evolution of the exercise is tightly managed. This can be a very thorough way of testing specific aspects but may not evaluate whether a plan is sufficiently flexible to deal with the unexpected.

- **Free play**

  Free play exercises are much more spontaneous. Once the opening scenario has been established, the participants' actions dictate subsequent events. This requires a large directing staff, a comprehensive scenario and access to much more background information. Although these can be stimulating in terms of realism and having to cope with the unexpected, it is possible that whole areas of a plan which require validation may be bypassed.

- **Or a combination of controlled and free play.**

7.3.3 Live exercise

Live exercises range from a small-scale test of one component of the response, like evacuation – ranging from a building or 'incident' site to an affected community – through to a full-scale test of the whole organisation's response to an incident. Live exercises provide the best means of confirming the satisfactory operation of emergency communications, and the use of 'casualties' can add to the realism. Live exercises provide the only means of testing fully the crucial arrangements for handling the media (Home Office 1998).

The objectives for a live exercise may include:

- activating and testing the plan under 'live' conditions
- identifying 'bottlenecks' within the Trust
- exercising the organisation and management of the control room
- exercising key locations identified in the plan, e.g. room for relatives and friends.

Key aspects of a live exercise:

- Setting a realistic time frame for planning and completing the exercise.
- Forming a planning group (one may already exist, e.g. Trust emergency planning group). Those involved in planning the exercise should not participate directly, but can participate as umpires or observers.

- The exercise planning group should agree whether there should be any prior publicity. It may be advisable to issue prior notification to members of the public in the vicinity of the exercise, to prevent any undue alarm.

- 'The safety of staff during live exercises is of paramount importance. In live exercises, all participants ... should be made aware of any hazards within the area and reminded of safety issues' (Home Office 1998).

- 'Exercises may be given a codename which should then be mandatory as a prefix to all messages – verbal or written – during the exercise' (Home Office 1998), e.g. 'Exercise Frontal Lobe' or 'Exercise Fluffy'.

- 'A codeword, which can be used to identify that a real incident has occurred and is not part of the exercise, should be agreed and circulated to all participants prior to the event. This could also be used if there are real casualties during the exercise' (Home Office 1998). An example of a commonly used codeword is 'No duff'.

- A 'hot' debrief (refer to Chapter 12 for further information on debriefing) of the participants must occur to ensure that any key issues, which urgently need to be resolved, can be raised. The exercise log, 'hot' debrief notes and directing staff notes should be used to compile a written report into the exercise, which should include a section on 'lessons identified'.

- Any lessons identified from the live exercise should be actioned and attached to any report. Copies of the report should be made available to the Trust's Chief Executive, Strategic Health Authority, sector/county EPLO (where in post) and RHEPA.

7.4 Summary

This chapter has outlined some of the key elements about planning training and exercises. Despite the requirement to plan for the required formal exercises and training, Trusts are encouraged to undertake regular, less-formal exercises to promote emergency planning as part of regular day-to-day work practices.

Box 7.4 Exercise checklist

1. Agree the scenario, extent and aim of the exercise with senior management as part of the exercise planning team (and multi-agency partners if participating).

2. Sketch out and then develop the main events of the exercise and associated timetables.

3. Determine and confirm the availability of the outside agencies to be involved, such as the media or voluntary agencies.

4. List the facilities required for the exercise and confirm their availability, e.g. transport, buildings and equipment.

5. Ensure that all communications to be used during the exercise have been tested at some stage prior to the exercise. Ahead of a live exercise, test radios, mobile phones, etc. in the locations in which they will be used, as near to the date of the exercise as possible.

6. Check that umpires and directing staff for each stage of the exercise are clearly identified and properly briefed.

7. If the exercise links a number of activities or functions which are dependent on each other, confirm that each has been individually tested beforehand.

8. Ensure that all participants have been briefed and ensure that all players are aware of the procedures to be followed if a real emergency occurs during the exercise.

9. If spectators are to be invited, including the media, ensure that they are clearly identified and properly marshalled, and arrange for them to be kept informed of the progress of the exercise. Ensure their safety.

10. For longer exercises, arrange catering and toilet facilities.

11. Warn the local media, emergency services switchboards/controls and any neighbours who might be worried or affected by the exercise. Position 'Exercise in Progress' signs if appropriate.

12. Ensure that senior management, directing staff, umpires and key players are aware of the time and location for the 'hot' debrief, and circulate a timetable for a full debrief.

13. Agree and prepare a detailed set of recommendations, each one accompanied by an action addressee and timescale.

14. Prepare a clear and concise summary report of the exercise to distribute to all participating organisations and groups, together with major recommendations.

15. Discuss with senior management the outcome of the exercise and agree the future exercise programme.

16. Thank all participants.

(Adapted from Home Office 1998)

7.5   Notes

1. Section 7.2 is reproduced from Department of Health (1998), with the kind permission of the Department of Health.

2. This information about types of exercises is reproduced with the kind permission of Crown Copyright 1998.

8

The Combined Response: an Integrated Approach to Major Incident Management

Jim Stuart-Black

8.1 Introduction

Most of this handbook focuses on the role of the emergency planner within the health economy. To fully understand the context within which the planner works, it is essential to understand the roles and responsibilities of a number of key agencies. At times, these agencies may be operating in support of a major incident declared by and affecting your own organisation alone, or, as will often be the case, you will be operating in support of other agencies as part of an overarching strategic framework.

The tragic events of 11 September 2001 not only heralded a new world order in geo-strategic terms, but also created a unique window of opportunity – indeed, something of a reformation within the world of emergency planning. British authorities have opened the doors to a full and frank review of emergency planning arrangements to respond to major incidents and potential catastrophic events. Catastrophic event planning, consequence and crisis management, horizon scanning and business continuity have become increasingly recognised as some of the new terms in emergency planning throughout the country – terms that all emergency planning practitioners must gain knowledge of.

Local planning groups, often chaired by the local authority, should meet on a regular basis to discuss arrangements for responding to major incidents. If such a group does not seem to exist, liaise with the local authority emergency planning officer to develop sound working practices.

These planning groups are not new in concept, although their content, focus and scale have increased exponentially. Groups no longer deal with just the traditional issues of flooding, train crashes and control of major accident hazards – they now address the complex issues caused by the perceived increase in the threat of chemical, biological, radiological and nuclear (CBRN) incidents, catastrophic incident management and so on.

A clear understanding of the roles and responsibilities of partner agencies, and the need to develop an integrated and harmonised approach to emergency planning, will ensure that you are able to develop robust plans.

8.2 Command, control and coordination

In order to achieve a combined and coordinated response to a major incident, the capabilities of the emergency services must be closely linked with those of local authorities and other agencies.[1] A generic management framework has been agreed nationally which embodies the same principles, irrespective of the cause or nature of the incident, but it remains flexible to individual circumstances. This framework:

- defines relationships between differing levels of management
- allows each agency to tailor its own response plans to interface with the plans of others

- ensures all parties involved understand their relative roles in the combined response
- retains sufficient flexibility of options to suit local circumstances.

Under the framework, the management of the response to major emergencies will normally be undertaken at one or more of three levels – **operational, tactical** and **strategic** (see Figure 8.1). The degree of management required will depend on the nature and scale of the emergency. It is a characteristic of the command and control chain that the management framework tends to be implemented from the bottom up.

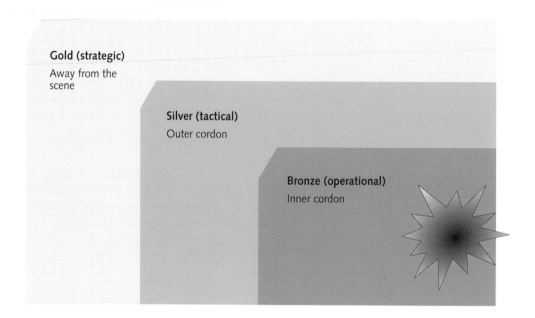

Figure 8.1 Scene management

The terms **Bronze**, **Silver** and **Gold** (for operational, tactical and strategic respectively) are in common use in many organisations as substitutes, e.g. 'Bronze commanders', 'Gold control'. They provide less clarity, however, for those unfamiliar with the topic. Interpretation of what they mean does vary and further confusion can arise if they are equated too closely with rank structures. The terms operational, tactical and strategic are therefore preferred in this publication as making clear the functions.

At the start of any incident for which there has been no warning, the operational level will be activated first. Either the escalation of the incident, or a greater awareness of the situation, may require the implementation of a tactical level and, finally, a strategic level should this prove necessary.

In its planning, each agency will need to recognise these three management levels and the functions they need to undertake. This will allow the integration of management processes across agency boundaries. It is not intended that the management levels necessarily predetermine the rank or seniority of the individual discharging the functions.

If any one agency activates its major incident plans (declares a major incident) then others need to assess their potential involvement and liaison arrangements in line with agreed protocols. It may or may not be necessary for others to start to activate their own major incident plan. The authority to declare a major incident for an organisation is vested in appropriate officers of that organisation. A major incident for one is not necessarily a major incident for others.

Operational level – BRONZE

The operational level of management reflects the normal day-to-day arrangements for responding to smaller scale emergencies. It is the level at which the management of 'hands-on' work is undertaken at the incident site(s) or associated areas.

First responders will take appropriate immediate measures and assess the extent of problems. There must be due regard to risk reduction measures and the health and safety of personnel. Operational commanders or managers will concentrate their resources on the specific tasks within their areas of responsibility. They will act on delegated responsibility from their parent organisations until other levels of command are established.

Individual agencies retain full command of the resources that they apply within a geographical area or use for a specific purpose. Each agency should liaise fully and continually with others to ensure an efficient and combined effort. The police will normally act as the coordinator of the response at an identifiable scene.

These arrangements will be adequate for the effective coordination and resolution of most minor emergencies. However, for more serious incidents that require significantly greater resources, it may be necessary to implement an additional level of management. A key function of an operational commander or manager will be to consider whether circumstances warrant a tactical level of management.

Tactical level – SILVER

A tactical level of management is introduced to provide overall management of the response. Tactical managers determine priorities in allocating resources, obtain further resources as required, and plan and coordinate when tasks will be undertaken. They must take appropriate risk reduction measures and give due regard to health and safety requirements.

Where there is an identifiable scene, tactical management is usually undertaken from an Incident Control Point established in the vicinity. Many tactical functions will then be discharged at or close to the scene. However, some agencies (for example, local authorities) will prefer to operate from their administrative offices, but will often send liaison officers to enhance coordination. Planning must also take into account that there may be a number of individual scenes, or in fact no particular scene to attend (for widespread disruption, health emergencies, or if the incident is overseas, etc.).

Inter-agency meetings at appropriate intervals between tactical managers and relevant liaison officers will aim to achieve effective coordination. Tactical managers must concentrate on overall general management. While they need to be aware of what is happening at operational level they should leave the responsibility for dealing with that level to operational managers. When the situation warrants it a strategic level of management/command should be established as early as possible.

Strategic level – GOLD

In exceptional circumstances, one or more agencies may find it necessary to implement a strategic level of management. Major emergencies can place considerable demands on the resources of the responding organisations, with consequent disruption to day-to-day activities. They may have long-term implications for people or the environment.

Such matters require attention by senior management (and possibly also by elected members in local authorities).

The purpose of implementing a strategic level of management is to establish a framework of policy within which tactical managers will work. Strategic managers will:

- establish a framework for the overall management of the incident

- determine strategic objectives that should be recorded and subject to regular review

- rapidly formulate and implement an integrated media policy

- ensure there are clear lines of communication with the tactical managers/commanders

- ensure there is long-term resourcing and expertise for management/command resilience

- give consideration to the prioritisation of demands from any number of tactical managers

- decide on what resources or expertise can be made available for tactical commander requirements

- undertake appropriate liaison with strategic managers in other agencies

- plan beyond the immediate response phase for recovering from the emergency and returning to a state of normality.

Strategic command for major incidents should be seen as standard practice, not the exception. It is easy to dismantle if not required, and removes the potential for tactical managers/commanders to be reluctant to ask for a strategic level of management/command. The need for a strategic level may arise if tactical management does not have the required resources or expertise available. It may also arise if there is a need to coordinate more than one incident/scene for which tactical command has been established. Strategic management is normally undertaken away from any major emergency scene.

The requirement for strategic management may be confined to one particular agency. However, certain incidents require a multi-agency response at the strategic level when the issues which arise affect the responsibilities or activities of more than one organisation. Experience has shown that such issues can best be dealt with by establishing a strategic coordinating group. This does not replace individual agencies' strategic management mechanisms, which will continue, but complements them to ensure that policy and approaches are effectively coordinated.

The Strategic Coordinating Group

It will normally be a police responsibility to establish and chair the Strategic Coordinating Group (SCG). However, due to the nature of some major incidents, other agencies may wish to initiate its formation and chair the group, e.g. for a rabies threat. Chairmanship may at some stage be passed to another agency (e.g. from the police to the local authority to manage the recovery phase). The Strategic Coordinating Group is normally made up from a nominated senior member from each statutory agency involved with the response. Each person must be able to make executive decisions in respect of resources within their agency, and each must have the authority to seek the aid of other agencies in support of their role.

The Strategic Coordinating Group should be based at an appropriate pre-planned location, away from the noise and confusion of the scene. It is usual to locate the

Strategic Coordination Group at police headquarters, but this may move to the local authority during the recovery phase, when the emergency services may have little or no involvement.

8.3 Agencies providing or contributing to the response

For sudden events, the emergency services, i.e. the police, fire, ambulance and coastguard services, maintain a state of readiness so that they can provide a rapid initial response and early alerting of local authorities and other services. All organisations that need to respond quickly to an emergency will have arrangements which can be activated at short notice. These arrangements should be clearly established and promulgated to all who may be involved in the response.

The emergency services, local authorities, government departments and other organisations, such as the utilities, voluntary organisations and faith communities, have produced single service (and sometimes single issue) planning documents. This publication draws on them to offer guidance on how the procedures and operations of each of the organisations involved can be combined and coordinated to provide an efficient and effective response.

At sudden-impact major emergencies which have an identifiable scene or scenes, each service or agency working at the scene(s) has its own particular roles and functions. Some of the key ones are described in the following sections.

The Police Service

The police will normally coordinate all the activities of those responding at and around the scene of a land-based emergency. The saving and protection of life is the priority, but as far as possible the scene must be preserved to provide evidence for subsequent enquiries and possibly criminal proceedings. Once life saving is complete, the area will be preserved as a scene of crime until it is established as otherwise (unless the emergency results from severe weather or other natural phenomena, and no element of human culpability is involved). Where practicable the police, in consultation with other emergency services and specialists, will establish and maintain cordons at appropriate distances. Cordons are established to facilitate the work of the other emergency services and support organisations in the saving of life, the protection of the public and the care of survivors. The primary areas of police responsibility at a major incident are:

- the saving of life, together with the other emergency services
- the coordination of the emergency services, local authorities and other organisations acting in support at the scene of the incident
- to secure, protect and preserve the scene and to control sightseers and traffic through the use of cordons
- the investigation of the incident and the obtaining and securing of evidence in conjunction with other investigative bodies where applicable
- the collection and distribution of casualty information
- the identification of the dead on behalf of Her Majesty's (HM) Coroner
- the prevention of crime
- family liaison, and
- short-term measures to restore normality after all necessary actions have been taken.

The Fire Service

The primary role of the Fire Service in a major emergency is the rescue of people trapped by fire, wreckage or debris. They will prevent further escalation of an incident by controlling or extinguishing fires, by rescuing people and by undertaking other protective measures. They will deal with released chemicals or other contaminants in order to render the incident site safe or recommend exclusion zones. They will also assist the Ambulance Service with casualty handling, and the Police Service with recovery of bodies.

The Fire Service is likely to take the lead on health and safety issues for personnel of all agencies working within the inner cordon. The Fire Service will manage access to the inner cordon under their Incident Command System, liaising with the police about who should be allowed access. It is expected that other agency workers attending the scene come issued with the appropriate level of personal protective equipment and that they are adequately trained and briefed. However, in the event of any situation which is, or which is suspected to be, the result of terrorism, police will assume overall control and take initial responsibility for safety management, but the main responsibility for rescuing people and saving lives remains with the Fire Service.

The primary areas of the Fire Service's responsibility at a major incident are:

- life saving through search and rescue

- fire fighting and fire prevention

- rendering humanitarian services

- management of hazardous materials and protecting the environment

- provision of qualified scientific advice in relation to HAZMAT incidents via their scientific advisers

- salvage and damage control

- safety management within the inner cordon, and

- maintaining emergency service cover throughout the brigade area and returning to a state of normal functioning at the earliest time.

The National Health Service

Section 9.5 of Chapter 9 gives further information on the roles and responsibilities of the NHS.

The Ambulance Service

Ambulance Services have responsibility for coordinating the on-site National Health Service response and determining the hospital(s) to which injured persons should be taken, which may depend on the types of injuries received. The Ambulance Incident Officer (AIO) is the officer of the Ambulance Service with overall responsibility for the service's work at the scene of a major incident. If necessary, the Ambulance Service will seek the attendance of a Medical Incident Officer (see Hospitals, below).

The Ambulance Service, in conjunction with the Medical Incident Officer and medical teams, endeavours to sustain life through effective emergency treatment at the scene, to determine the priority for release of trapped casualties and decontamination in conjunction with the Fire Service, and to transport the injured in order of priority to receiving hospitals.

The Ambulance Service may seek support from voluntary aid societies (British Red Cross, St. John Ambulance and St. Andrew's Ambulance) in managing and transporting casualties.

Hospitals

Hospitals with major accident and emergency departments have been designated as potential casualty-receiving hospitals. They respond to requests from the Ambulance Service to receive casualties for medical treatment and also provide appropriately trained staff to act as Mobile Medical Teams and Medical Incident Officers.

A Medical Incident Officer has overall responsibility (in close liaison with the Ambulance Incident Officer) for the management of medical resources at the scene of a major incident. He/she should not be a member of a Mobile Medical Team.

Other hospitals provide support to receiving hospitals by taking patient transfers, etc.

Public health

The NHS makes public health advice available to the emergency services, NHS organisations and the public on a 24-hour basis. This advice is crucial for the control of communicable diseases and for public health concerns relating to hazards in chemical, biological, radiological and nuclear incidents.

Primary and community care services

The provision of primary and community care support is a crucial aspect of the NHS response. These services cover a range of health professions including general practitioners (GPs), community nurses, health visitors, mental health services and pharmacists, many of whom would need to be involved following a major incident. Primary Care Trusts (PCTs) should therefore be involved in emergency planning processes.

HM Coroner

The role of the coroner is defined by statute. Coroners have responsibilities in relation to bodies lying within their district of those who have met a violent or unnatural death, or a sudden death of unknown cause. They have to determine who has died, how, and when and where the death came about. This function is regardless of whether or not the cause of death arose within their district. They normally undertake this duty at a formal inquest (though if the incident results in a public inquiry chaired by a judge, a full inquest may not be held).

Coroners should have an emergency plan relating to multiple fatalities, and coroners' officers should be familiar with its content. They should also be familiar with the police major incident plan for their own area and with the local authority emergency plan.

The powers and duties of coroners do not vary with the number of people who are killed or the circumstances in which the deaths occur. A body at the scene of an incident should not be moved without the authority of the coroner, and only the coroner may authorise a post-mortem and the release of a body to relatives. In general, the police act as the coroner's officers when dealing with fatalities arising from an incident.

HM Coastguard Agency

The primary responsibility of HM Coastguard is to initiate and coordinate civil maritime search and rescue within the United Kingdom Search and Rescue Region

(UKSRR). Local coastal safety committees, based on police force boundaries, ensure effective coordination of resources between police and coastguard for land-based incidents on or adjacent to coastlines.

The Marine Pollution Control Unit is responsible for dealing with pollution at sea and, in conjunction with local authorities, for the shoreline clean-up.

Local authorities

Each local authority manages a civil contingency planning function. Civil protection (or emergency planning) personnel act as a hub to coordinate the planning, training and exercising within local authority departments. The effectiveness of this hub is fundamental to the discharge of related community responsibilities in an emergency, whatever the cause.

Local authority planning is carried out in close cooperation with the emergency services, utilities, many other industrial and commercial organisations, central government departments such as the Ministry of Defence or Department of Health, other statutory organisations such as the Environment Agency, and many voluntary agencies.

The principal concern of local authorities in the immediate aftermath of an emergency is to provide support for the people in their area. Generally, they do so by cooperating in the first instance with the emergency services in the overall response.

However, they also have many specific responsibilities of their own. They will use the resources of local authority departments to mitigate the effects of emergencies on people, property and infrastructure, and play a key role in coordinating the response from the voluntary sector. They also endeavour to continue to provide [business as usual] support and care for the local and wider community throughout any disruption.

As part of the local response, plans should already have been agreed for opening additional spaces at existing public or NHS mortuaries and/or establishing temporary mortuaries. These plans should include how to locate staff.

As the emphasis moves in time from immediate response to recovery, the local authority will take a leading role to facilitate the rehabilitation of the community and restoration of the environment. Even a relatively small emergency may overwhelm the resources of the local authority in whose area it occurs. Against this possibility plans need to be made which will, in appropriate circumstances, trigger arrangements for mutual aid from neighbouring authorities, delivering cross-boundary assistance if required. Arrangements may range from simple agreements offering whatever assistance is available in the event of an incident to more formal arrangements for the shared use of resources. This could include the use of vehicles, equipment and people. (Payment arrangements may need to be included in any agreement.)

Regional Resilience Teams

London Resilience was the first Regional Resilience Team created within the Civil Contingencies Secretariat (Norman 2002). Having been established after the events of 11 September 2001, the London team (once viewed as a temporary subcommittee), tasked with assessing the state of 'resilience' of emergency management within the capital, is a critical part of the London planning arrangements. The team is still largely staffed by individuals seconded from agencies, including among others the Metropolitan Police, London Ambulance Service and local authorities. Owing to the success of the London team, the concept of Regional Resilience Teams has been expanded throughout England and Wales, and now fulfils a critical role.

Volunteers

Bona fide volunteers can contribute to a wide range of activities, either as members of a voluntary organisation or as individuals. They will always be under the control of a statutory authority.

8.4 Objectives for a combined response

Irrespective of the particular responsibilities of organisations and agencies who may be involved with the disaster response, they will all work to the following common objectives:

- saving and protecting life
- relieving suffering
- protecting property
- providing the public with information
- containing the emergency – limiting its escalation or spread
- maintaining critical services
- maintaining normal services at an appropriate level
- protecting the health and safety of personnel
- safeguarding the environment
- facilitating investigations and inquiries
- promoting self-help and recovery
- restoring normality as soon as possible
- evaluating the response and identifying lessons to be learned.

8.5 Roles and responsibilities in the event of a CBRN incident

Refer to Figure 10.1 for a diagrammatic representation of the on-scene response.[2]

The Police Service

The Police Service will:

- be responsible for the overall coordination of the emergency response to any incident
- take initial responsibility for safety management within the inner cordon at terrorist incidents
- agree the boundary of the inner cordon with the Fire Service and determine the boundary of the outer cordon, subject to the best scientific and other inter-agency advice available
- until it is determined otherwise, treat the site as a crime scene, maintain the integrity of the scene and cordons, ensure that people who are unprotected by appropriate level PPE do not enter the inner cordon, and ensure that, where the contamination is the result of a suspected criminal act, correct evidence collection, labelling, sealing, storage and recording procedures are carried out in respect of property
- identify and supervise a safe holding place for this property and be responsible for deciding at what point it may be safe to return it to its owners

- liaise with the coroner
- provide hospital security and documentation team(s) – in PPE if appropriate
- decide whether to seek military assistance
- in consultation with the local authority, establish and staff friends and relatives reception centres at suitable locations.

The Fire Service

The Fire and Rescue Service will:

- carry out scene assessment in consultation with the police
- perform urban search and rescue
- in consultation with the police, establish an inner cordon and determine initial access arrangements
- coordinate hazard assessment (also in consultation with the police)
- within the terms of the Memorandum of Understanding between the Office of the Deputy Prime Minister and the Department of Health (and equivalent agreements or protocols in the devolved administrations), work with the Ambulance Service to provide a mass decontamination service
- in accordance with locally agreed arrangements, assist the ambulance and health services in providing casualty decontamination
- take responsibility for safety management within the inner cordon
- supply fire service personnel with PPE and equipment for activity inside the inner cordon
- assist with the mitigation of the effects of hazardous materials
- minimise the impact on the environment during the emergency phase of an incident, in liaison with the Environment Agency (and equivalent authorities in the devolved administrations).

The Ambulance Service

The Ambulance Service[3] will:

- coordinate all health service activities on site
- assume responsibility for casualty decontamination – requesting Fire Service assistance where required
- decontaminate other victims together with the Fire Service in accordance with the Memorandum of Understanding between the Office of the Deputy Prime Minister and the Department of Health (and equivalent agreements or protocols in the devolved administrations)
- treat and reassure any patients or potential patients at the scene
- notify the relevant Accident and Emergency departments that a CBRN incident has occurred and advise of the potential for self-presenting patients
- arrange the provision of clinical advice and assistance to support on-site decontamination
- wherever possible, provide limited patient triage and treatment at the inner cordon prior to decontamination
- provide subsequent assessment, treatment and patient transport.

The National Health Service and the Health Protection Agency

The National Health Service (NHS) and Health Protection Agency (HPA) will:

- liaise with the Ambulance Service about the level of resources needed as a result of the incident

- where practicable, provide a site medical officer to liaise with the emergency services, oversee the medical countermeasures at the scene and make arrangements for the certification of death

- at the request of the Police Incident Commander, or where there is otherwise sufficient cause, set up a Joint Health Advisory Cell (JHAC)[4] to offer advice to the multi-agency strategic coordination group about public health issues, including information which is suitable for distribution to the public

- monitor the health of all responders and those affected, and implement measures to ensure the general public are kept informed and as safe as possible

- provide medical assistance and follow-up advice at survivor reception centres and holding areas, to treat, monitor and reassure casualties (including those who self-present)

- liaise with the Food Standards Agency (FSA), the Environment Agency or SEPA on all relevant aspects of the release of contaminant

- monitor the symptoms of people self-presenting at hospitals and GPs' surgeries, to ensure that medical evidence of biological releases is identified as quickly as possible

- monitor the medium- and long-term health of those in affected communities as part of the recovery process.

The Environment Agency and Scottish Environmental Protection Agency

The Environment Agency (EA)/Scottish Environmental Protection Agency (SEPA) will:

- assess the risk posed by the incident to the environment, helping to identify where material might disperse to via environmental pathways, and who and what might be at risk and, where practicable, giving advice about the location of decontamination facilities

- in cases where flushed materials and contaminated waters cannot reasonably be contained and stored, identify the watercourses and drainage systems at risk and warn water companies, water abstractors and relevant local authorities

- make staff available at command centres to assist the continuing hazard and risk assessments

- help the emergency services to identify facilities and contractors for the storage, transport and disposal of contaminated waters or solid waste materials

- where appropriate, investigate breaches of environmental regulation and report these for consideration of prosecution

- support the emergency services, local authorities, water companies and the Food Standards Agency in dealing with environmental issues.

The local authority

The local authority will:

- organise, staff and provide logistical support at survivor reception centres, to accommodate people who have been decontaminated at the scene and who, while not requiring acute hospital treatment, need short-term shelter, first aid, interview and documentation

- organise, staff and provide logistical support at rest centres for the temporary accommodation of evacuees, with overnight facilities where appropriate and invoking mutual aid arrangements with neighbouring authorities if necessary

- in consultation with the police, establish and staff friends and relatives reception centres

- lead the work of voluntary agencies in response to the incident

- lead the recovery phase.

8.6 Summary

This chapter has provided the multi-agency content for emergency planning by outlining key roles and responsibilities and the frameworks used to provide a harmonised approach to emergency planning. It is vital that these relationships are captured within your planning process to ensure integrated and robust plans.

8.7 Notes

1. Sections 8.2 to 8.5 have been adapted from Home Office (2003) and Cabinet Office (2003), with kind permission from Crown Copyright. Information has also been reproduced from LESLP (2003), with the kind permission of the Metropolitan Police Service.

2. Section 8.5 has been reproduced from the Home Office (2004) publication, *The Decontamination of People Exposed to Chemical, Biological, Radiological or Nuclear (CBRN) Substances or Material: Strategic National Guidance*, with the kind permission of Crown Copyright. See Chapter 10 of this handbook for further detail on the roles and responsibilities in the event of CBRN incidents.

3. For further information on the roles and responsibilities of the Ambulance Service, see Chapter 9.

4. It is understood at the time of writing that the term JHAC was being reviewed and was likely to be renamed Health Advice Team (HAT). To reflect the arrangements at the time of writing, reference is made to JHAC in a number of chapters in this handbook.

9

The Health Response: Roles and Responsibilities

Sarah Norman

9.1 Introduction

In order to promote a National Health Service and Health Protection Agency response that meshes together seamlessly from local to national level, it is important to understand the roles, responsibilities and relationships of those organisations within the health-care economy that play a vital role in the response to major incidents. This chapter will outline these roles and responsibilities.

During the writing of this handbook, the Department of Health was reviewing the document *Planning for Major Incidents* (1998). Although it was recognised the review may affect the roles and responsibilities of a number of health organisations, at the time of writing this handbook, the new Department of Health Publication, *The NHS Emergency Planning Guidance* (2005), had not been released.

9.2 The Department of Health: Operational Doctrine

The following section sets out the Department of Health's Operational Doctrine for handling major incidents,[1] which includes:

- the basic doctrine
- the chain of command
- incidents that impact upon the capacity or continuity of NHS services
- incidents that threaten the wider health of the community.

Basic doctrine

It is in the nature of major incidents that they are unpredictable, and each will present a unique set of challenges. Our task is not to anticipate them in detail. It is to have a set of expertise available and to have developed a set of core processes to handle the uncertainty and unpredictability of whatever happens.

Given the objective stated above, our basic doctrine can be seen as comprising:

- **speed and flexibility** at local operational level, delivered by hospitals, Ambulance Services, and primary care providers (local Trusts) and, where necessary, by public health practitioners
- **active mutual aid** across organisational boundaries coordinated by the Strategic Health Authority (SHA) or the Primary Care Trust (PCT) leading the response
- a strong **central capability** to oversee and support SHAs at the Department of Health (DH).

The first priority is to stress the importance of ensuring that staff who will be called upon to deliver services during an incident have maximum local freedom to adapt and develop responses to an uncertain and complex environment.

In some situations local staff will need assistance from neighbours. This requires greater inter-operability, standardisation of equipment, training and systems, and more vigorous coordination by SHAs. The SHAs must take a proactive lead in guaranteeing the availability of practical mutual aid and support both within their area and across SHA boundaries.

Local plans should be drawn up in conjunction with social care and other partners, and with a clear understanding that the Department of Health will put in place a central contingency team whenever the need arises. This central 'ops room' capability will be specifically to coordinate and support the work of SHAs – not to disempower local decision-makers – and to provide the link into the wider machinery of government at national level.

Each part of the health and social care system has a role to play. Every organisation needs to understand not only its own responsibilities, but also those of others that will support and complement its own efforts.

The chain of command

Major disruptive challenges or large-scale incidents may impact upon health care in two main ways:

(a) The incident/occurrence itself or its aftermath might rapidly threaten the capacity or continuity of health service provision. Large-scale accidents, terrorist incidents or threats to the supply chain would be examples.

(b) The incident/occurrence – or its consequences – may not have a rapid impact on health services but may threaten the wider health of the community – either immediately or at some subsequent stage. Outbreaks of infectious diseases, food contamination or water or air pollution are examples.

The speed and unpredictability with which these incidents can develop is such that it is essential to have crystal-clear arrangements for coordination, command and control. In the former type of incident that responsibility will naturally fall to SHAs, PCTs and those NHS organisations providing the front-line response. In the latter, the Regional Director of Public Health and the public health function would have the specialist knowledge and experience required to provide advice. In each case the Health Protection Agency would also have a critical role in providing advice and operational support.

However, it has to be recognised that some incidents may have both characteristics from the outset – or that the characteristics may change as the incident develops. It is therefore essential that local plans and structures are harmonised and that the NHS management and public health aspects are approached in a fully collaborative way.

Incidents impacting upon the capacity or continuity of NHS services

In the initial phase of any incident immediately affecting the NHS, the Ambulance Service in whose area it occurs will coordinate and control all NHS resources deployed to the scene – unless on health service premises. The Ambulance Incident Officer (Silver or Bronze) will ensure that the NHS response is coordinated and focused, that adequate resources are deployed, and that communication channels are established. Depending on the type and duration, the on-site health coordination role might pass to other health specialists as the incident develops.

PCTs will mobilise primary and community care resources to support acute hospital provision and to sustain those needing care at home, including accessing social care support. They must also take steps to monitor and safeguard the health of the local population for the duration of an incident, and be capable of quickly disseminating health advice to the public if required. The HPA will provide support and contribute through its local health protection teams.

The SHA will coordinate the overall response and all local aspects of NHS support for the incident within its boundary, and be responsible for activating links across SHA boundaries and with social care agencies. Support and advice will be available from the Regional Directors of Public Health and the HPA's local and regional health protection teams.

Incidents that threaten the wider health of the community

For any emergency where the immediate impact is likely to be mainly on public health rather than the day-to-day operation of the NHS, responsibility for overall health coordination and control will rest with the Regional Director of Public Health or nominated representative at PCT or SHA level. They will have the support and expertise of the HPA and its regional health protection teams available, and can also provide a liaison link to Regional Offices of Government. SHAs will coordinate NHS responses as required.

9.3 The Department of Health: the health response at national level

The Department of Health has an overall responsibility to ensure that the NHS is adequately prepared for major incidents. This means that it should be confident that plans are in place, validated and tested, and that adequate resources are available to ensure that plans can be activated effectively should the need arise. However, it also has a coordinating role, and in the event of a major incident which either impacts over a number of Strategic Health Authority (SHA) areas and/or is of regional or national significance, the Department of Health will establish a coordination centre to act as the link between the NHS and wider government. As part of communication arrangements, there must be direct reporting capability between SHAs and the Department of Health. The Operational Doctrine provides the following direction for incidents requiring national coordination:

- Although there are public health links to government offices for the regions, the NHS does not have a regional management structure. If the scale of an incident escalates beyond the local SHA's capacity or area, or its duration or nature is such that wider NHS resources are required, the Department of Health will implement national coordinating arrangements. Those arrangements are intended to support the SHA, ensure that wider NHS resources are made available and that wider government assistance is accessed if required.

- Overall accountability is depicted in Figure 9.1. There may need to be local variation in the way in which these responsibilities are discharged, but it is essential that clearly agreed escalation triggers and mechanisms are contained in each local plan.

The Department of Health is responsible for a number of functions, which include:

- overall coordination of the national health response, including the media lead at national level

- response to activation of arrangements at national level such as Reception Arrangements for Military Patients (RAMP)

- lead government department for communicable or infectious diseases

- briefing for ministers and Chief Medical Officer

- liaison across government

- Department of Health representation at Cabinet Office Briefing Room (COBR)

- policy development

- international liaison, including overseas forward planning (Department of Health 2004).

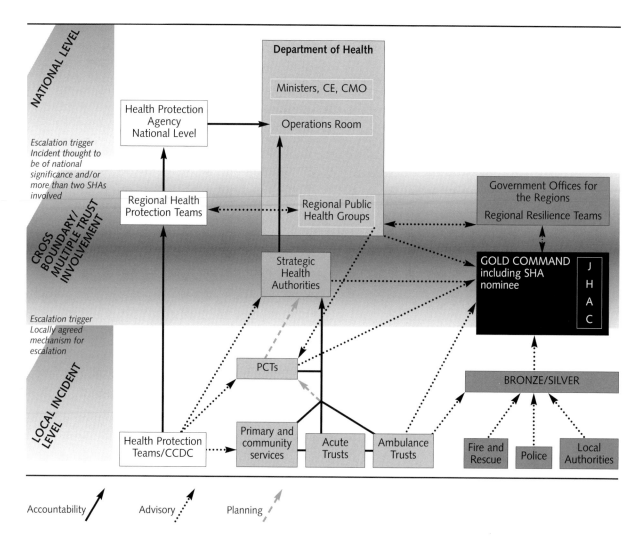

Figure 9.1 Accountabilities, planning and advisory roles for health organisations

Box 9.1 Obligations in the Operational Doctrine for the Department of Health

The Doctrine (Department of Health 2004) states:

The Department of Health will be responsible for national oversight and monitoring of all incidents that result in activation of a major incident plan. This does not mean it will necessarily always be involved in all of them – most will be handled at local or SHA level. It will whenever necessary – either when more than one SHA is substantially affected or when an incident has a 'national' characteristic – establish a national 'ops room' to support SHA management of incidents, to promote and encourage mutual aid and to act as focal point for links across Government.

9.4 The Health Protection Agency

The Chief Medical Officer for Health, Sir Liam Donaldson, announced the need for the Health Protection Agency in his report, *Getting Ahead of the Curve*, published in January 2002, which recognised the need to bring together the skills and expertise of a number of organisations to work in a more coordinated way to reduce the burden and consequences of health protection threats or disease (Department of Health 2002b). This would provide a more comprehensive and effective response to threats to the public's health. The Health Protection Agency's role involves:

- advising government on public health protection policies and programmes

- delivering services and supporting the NHS and other agencies to protect people from infectious diseases, poisons and chemical and radiological hazards

- providing an impartial and authoritative source of information and advice to professionals and the public

- responding to new threats to public health

- providing a rapid response to health protection emergencies, including the deliberate release of biological, chemical, poisonous or radioactive substances

- improving knowledge of health protection through research, development, education and training (Department of Health 2004).

In a response to a major incident, the Health Protection Agency will at national level provide:

- support to the Department of Health, including COBR

- public health response for the Department of Health and the NHS

- activation and coordination of the Health Protection Agency multi-division response

- expert input to the Joint Health Advisory Cell

- contact arrangements for clinicians (local, regional and national)

- coordination and provision of advice to the Department of Health, NHS, other government departments and the general public

- advice to devolved administrations on operational issues

- coordination and release of medical countermeasures and equipment

- preparatory measures for conventional major incidents (Department of Health 2004).

Box 9.2 Obligations in the Operational Doctrine for the Health
Protection Agency

The Doctrine (Department of Health 2004) states:

Health Protection Agency will provide specialist health emergency advice to the Department of Health, NHS and Regional Public Health Group. They will provide both advice and capacity to deal with communicable diseases and chemical incidents, and will work with the NRPB [now known as Radiological Protection Division] to create similar capability for nuclear and radiological incidents.

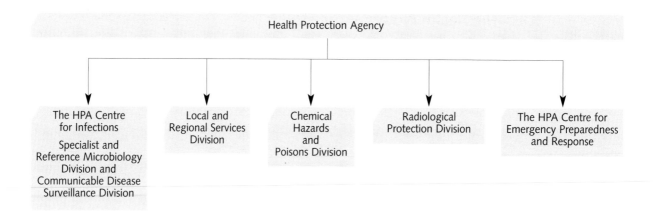

Figure 9.2 Divisions of the Health Protection Agency

The Health Protection Agency consists of five divisions (see Figure 9.2), which are able to operate at local, regional or national level. The roles and responsibilities of the five divisions are described below.

9.4.1 The Health Protection Agency Centre for Emergency Preparedness and Response

Emergencies, outbreaks of disease and chemical incidents have the potential to cause disruption for communities on a large scale and present operational problems to the NHS. Because disease outbreaks and chemical incidents can develop very rapidly, preparation and emergency planning are essential in order to minimise the impact on the public. Responding effectively means organisations working together to minimise the impact and achieve a return to normality as quickly as possible.

The Emergency Preparedness and Response Centre's roles include:

- Improving the speed and effectiveness of our overall response, both locally and nationally, in the event of any future incident or threat. This includes providing positive and authoritative messages about health protection measures in order to reduce public anxiety.

- Providing a central source of authoritative scientific/medical information and other specialist advice on both the planning and operational responses to major incidents and wider public health or other emergencies.

The Emergency Preparedness and Response Centre's areas of focus include:

- building on the existing major incident plans
- developing the infrastructure for surveillance and early recognition of events
- continuing to produce guidance for health protection for these new hazards
- identifying specific countermeasures and making sure they are available quickly
- providing training and testing new plans
- coordinating the Health Protection Agency's divisions and expertise in emergency situations (Department of Health 2004).

9.4.2 Local and Regional Services Division

The Local and Regional Services (LaRS) Division is based on nine regional teams, each with an epidemiologist, a microbiologist, Regional Health Emergency Planning

Adviser(s) and information staff. There are also 42 local protection teams, each with a consultant in communicable disease control. The role of the LaRS Division includes:

- supporting the Regional Director of Public Health in managing the response to major incidents and coordinating the local health protection teams

- giving specialist advice and support to PCTs, Acute Trusts and SHAs

- coordination of the response with other LAS teams in the regions and with the Department of Health

- long-term support following an incident by undertaking case follow-up, surveillance and monitoring as required.

The division's public health responsibilities include:

- taking a lead in managing the public health and environmental consequences of the event

- continually monitoring health within the population to detect events when they occur

- notifying/alerting agencies and sensitive populations, who may be unaware of the event or its potential consequences

- ensuring the provision of health care (NHS) and advice (Regional Public Health Cadre/JHAC) to manage the event and treat those affected, including to those responding to the incident

- identifying candidate agent(s) on advice from Regional Public Health Cadres/JHACs

- formulating case definitions

- active case finding and site visits, if appropriate

- investigation of cases, including microbiology and toxicology

- data collection of cases and database management

- dissemination of best available advice on clinical management from the Regional Public Health Cadre/JHAC to all health professionals, including environmental health

- working with police to exchange information on joint investigations, if necessary

- ensuring adequate health protection measures are implemented, on advice from Regional Public Health Cadres

- ensuring immediate actions are taken to manage the risk, including decontamination

- ensuring that health service resources are notified and protected

- epidemiological follow-up and health-care provision for those affected, including responders/health-care staff

- coordination of remediation activity to redress health and environment issues

- assessing the impact of the event on public health and the environment

- linking in with occupational health departments for affected responders and businesses

- organising and providing sampling and provision of countermeasures/medications

- mobilisation of resources (staff, equipment, medications) to meet demand

- enacting statutory legislation to effect actions (i.e. quarantine)

- signposting the public (and responders) to access appropriate health-care resources
- executing proper officer duties
- checking essential actions undertaken by responders to address risks to health and the environment.

Box 9.3 Obligations in the Operational Doctrine for Regional Public Health Groups

The Doctrine (Department of Health 2004) states:

Regional Public Health Groups led by Regional Directors of Public Health will ensure a 24-hour capability to support both the SHAs and the rest of the Department of Health, and where necessary to coordinate public health resources in responding to public health emergencies. The RDsPH will provide the health link to Regional Resilience mechanisms and act as the regional nominated coordinator in public health emergencies.

9.4.3 Chemical Hazards and Poisons Division

The role of the Chemical Hazards and Poisons (CHAPs) Division includes:

- giving advice, support and training for chemical incidents
- providing information and support to NHS and health professionals on toxicology
- surveillance of chemical hazards and their health effects
- maintaining the National Poisons database and National Poisons Information Service.

9.4.4 The Health Protection Agency Centre for Infections

The Health Protection Agency Centre for Infections has been created by combining the Specialist and Reference Microbiology Division (SRMD) and the Communicable Disease Surveillance Centre (CDSC). These two agencies have been replaced with the Communicable Disease Surveillance Division and the Specialist and Reference Microbiology Services Division.

Communicable Disease Surveillance Division

The role of the Communicable Disease Surveillance Division includes:

- coordinating the surveillance, alerting and response functions to infectious diseases in England
- coordination of control measures in cases of multi-regional outbreaks or incidents
- providing training programmes for those involved in the surveillance and control of infectious diseases
- providing a comprehensive public health information service for infectious diseases
- contributing to national policy development by the Department of Health and other government departments
- undertaking research and development to support the above public health responsibilities
- working with other national bodies to provide UK-wide protection against communicable diseases.

Specialist and Reference Microbiological Services Division

The role of the Specialist and Reference Microbiological Services Division includes:

- supporting a network of reference laboratories for microbiology
- the provision of specialist expertise and advice to hospitals and regional laboratories
- offering support for consultants in communicable disease control
- the provision of specialist tests not undertaken in other laboratories
- the provision of microbiological epidemiology and forensic microbiology.

9.4.5 Radiological Protection Division

The role of the Radiological Protection Division (RPD) includes:

- a requirement to provide formal advice on radiological protection standards for emergencies
- providing information and advice to government departments and agencies operations
- providing senior advisers at key locations, such as the Nuclear Emergency Briefing Room (NEBR) and Department of Health
- advising the Government Technical Adviser (GTA)/Military or Ministry of Defence Coordinating Authority (MCA), JHAC and local emergency centre (LEC)
- acting as senior spokesperson to the LEC media briefing centre
- the national coordination of monitoring resources
- the assessment of consequences
- the coordination of national arrangements for incidents involving radioactivity (NAIR).

9.5 The National Health Service

The NHS response involves a number of health organisations at local level, county/sector level and regional level, which work closely with the Local and Regional Services (LaRS) Division of the Health Protection Agency to provide an integrated health response to major incidents. As there is significant regional variation throughout England for the activation and coordination of these services in major incidents, only a broad indication will be given as to how the different levels interact.

The response role of the following services (refer to Figure 9.3) will be described in this section.

Local level:

- Acute Trusts
- Ambulance Trusts
- Primary Care Trusts (PCTs)
- Non-Acute Trusts such as Mental Health Trusts and Specialist Trusts (e.g. Great Ormond Street Hospital Trust).

County/sector level:

- lead PCTs
- SHAs.

Regional level:

- SHAs – which may provide a regional response through an on-call rota of SHA chief executives.

This section provides an overview of the roles and responsibilities of the individual Trusts and organisations that form the National Health Service.

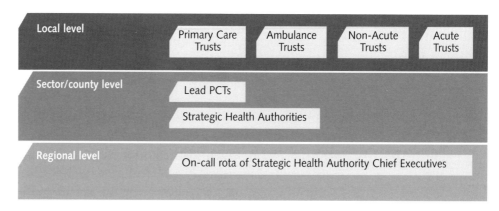

Figure 9.3 NHS organisations at local, sector/county and regional levels

9.5.1 The Acute Trust

The roles and responsibilities of Acute Trusts in a major incident are:

- to provide general supportive health care to casualties (both victims and responders)
- to liaise with the Ambulance Service, other hospitals and agencies in order to manage the impact of the incident
- to maintain communications with relatives and friends of existing patients and those from the incident, the local community, the media and very important persons (VIPs)
- to provide on-site medical care and advice
- to ensure the hospital continues all its essential functions
- to provide limited decontamination facilities and personal protective equipment (PPE) to manage contaminated self-presenting casualties (Department of Health 1998).

9.5.2 The Ambulance Trust

In a major incident which has a sudden onset and in which there are, or are likely to be, multiple casualties, the Ambulance Service's key roles are to:

- assess the incident
- coordinate the on-site operational response

- liaise with other emergency services on site
- identify and activate the resources needed to respond
- manage the NHS activity at the scene
- coordinate NHS communications at the scene
- treat casualties: assist extrication, triage, stabilise, and give initial treatment
- transport casualties to hospital
- protect the health and safety of all health service personnel on site
- undertake clinical decontamination of casualties at the scene if required
- maintain emergency and routine cover (Department of Health 1998).

Box 9.4 Obligations in the Operational Doctrine for hospitals and Ambulance Service Trusts

The Doctrine (Department of Health 2004) states:

All hospital and ambulance services trusts are responsible for deploying the right health-care resources to care for casualties either at the scene or at a hospital site. Each must be able to mobilise local resources flexibly and to the maximum extent consistent with maintaining essential care. Each trust must also plan to offer effective support to any neighbouring service that is substantially affected, and in return should be able to rely on such mutual support if it is needed.

9.5.3 Non-Acute Trusts (Mental Health Trusts or Specialist Trusts)

In a major incident the roles and responsibilities of Non-Acute Trusts include:

- support for Acute Trusts through the transfer of casualties (where appropriate)
- access to additional resources
- working with PCTs and the community to support the recovery phase
- linking with PCTs and the sector in coordinating services
- ensuring that patients involved in the incident are discharged home with appropriate support in the community
- continuing to provide core business services.

9.5.4 Primary Care Trusts

The roles and responsibilities of PCTs in major incidents include:

- coordinating the primary care, community and mental health response
- the delivery of primary and community health services through:
  o mobilisation of community resources
  o support of the NHS infrastructure for hospitals by enabling increased hospital capacity through avoiding admission and caring for early discharges
- assessing the impact on health and health services of every potential major incident
- treatment of minor casualties at minor injury centres, walk-in centres and general practices

- providing care and advice to evacuees, survivors and relatives, including replacement medication

- assisting acute hospitals by providing staff where appropriate and supporting accelerated discharge

- administration of prophylaxis, vaccines and countermeasures

- providing support, advice and leadership to the local community on health aspects of an incident

- working with the local authority and community to support the recovery phase

- ensuring that the services of all providers of health care are supported to meet the needs of the local population

- providing a strategic view on long-term threats (Department of Health 2002c).

Box 9.5 Obligations in the Operational Doctrine for Primary Care Trusts

The Doctrine (Department of Health 2004) states:

All Primary Care Trusts must be able to mobilise and direct health-care resources to local hospitals at short notice, to support them and to sustain patients in the community should these hospital services be reduced or compromised for a period. They must also plan to harness and effectively utilise primary care resources where needed ... for example by setting up ad hoc emergency assessment facilities or emergency vaccination programmes. They must also have agreed systems in place to enable them to work as 'lead' PCT with others or – as appropriate – in support of the 'lead' PCT.

9.5.5 Lead PCTs

Additional roles and responsibilities for lead PCTs during major incidents include:

- acting on behalf of 'linked' PCTs

- representing other PCTs in multi-agency planning, including liaison with police and local authorities

- coordination of own and other PCT plans across local police boundaries

- coordination of health and social care economy, operational and public health response (Department of Health 2002c: 5).

There are a number of differences in London:

- PCTs are almost all coterminous with London boroughs, each of which has its own emergency planning group which the local PCT will attend

- representation at police Gold control is undertaken by the SHA Chief Executive on an on-call rota basis

- the lead PCTs form part of the sector coordinating team with the SHA and Local Health Protection (see section 9.4.2).

9.5.6 Strategic Health Authorities

SHAs are the local headquarters of the NHS. As such, they will be able to mobilise and commit resources across the authority area, and will be responsible for the coordination of health services in the event of a major incident. SHAs are ultimately responsible to the Department of Health for the robustness of the plans of organisations within their area and that of the mutual aid components of the plans. SHAs need to demonstrate leadership across their area. SHAs need to be assured that plans are compatible and that mutual aid arrangements are in place and executable, which is particularly important across organisational boundaries.

SHAs should also ensure that appropriate and robust links are made with other organisations, including emergency services, local authorities, voluntary organisations and private-sector providers. These links must be regularly tested.

SHAs must be able to establish a management control team within two hours of the notification of an incident, and they must be able to communicate with every local NHS Trust. This should include a representative of the PCT(s) involved. There must be explicit reporting arrangements with all NHS bodies and with others, which can be sustained on a 24/7 basis for the duration of the incident. In some regions the SHA response forms the basis for the sector or county coordinating teams, while in other regions the SHA may operate as a single entity.

Box 9.6 Obligations in the Operational Doctrine for Strategic Health Authorities

The Doctrine (Department of Health 2004) states:

Each Strategic Health Authority must be able to guarantee strategic control of any incident that affects or seems likely to affect several hospitals or have a significant impact on primary care. Every SHA must ensure that the NHS within its area has unequivocal command and control structures, that escalation triggers and mechanisms are clearly described and understood, that escalation policies are clearly described, that capacity plans are available and that links within the NHS, with neighbouring SHAs, with Regional Directors of Public Health, the HPA and across into other sectors – including social care – are effective and durable. As part of this many SHAs will have 'lead' PCTs to work with.

9.5.7 County arrangements/sector coordinating teams

The county/sector arrangements are flexible in relation to local arrangements, and will differ between regions, but some of the more general roles and responsibilities at either county or sector level are:

- coordinating the overall response of the health and social care economy within the sector/county, working with the regional team and neighbouring sectors/counties
- notifying those NHS organisations who are not already alerted
- assessing the ongoing situation and identifying emerging issues
- providing resources to support the local effort using mutual and regional aid.

9.6 The Regional Health Emergency Planning Advisers

The Regional Health Emergency Planning Advisers (RHEPAs) located within each of the regions in England (with RHEPAs also in Wales, Scotland and Northern Ireland) are dedicated to providing health emergency planning advice, facilitation and support to a range of health organisations as well as multi-agency partners. The RHEPAs hold a unique position within the health-care economy: having joined the Health Protection Agency, they form the vital link between the NHS and the Health Protection Agency in ensuring continued focus on emergency preparedness. The roles and responsibilities of the RHEPAs are extensive (although there are regional differences), but generally they include the following:

- Advising on the preparation of plans and preparedness for the health economy.

- Actively contributing to the formulation of national, regional and local policies and strategies, contingency guidance and plans.

- Liaising with partner agencies and organisations at local, regional, governmental and national level.

- Providing a holistic systems approach to emergency planning within the national resilience framework. (Refer also to Chapter 8 for information about the regional resilience teams.)

- Ensuring that regional command and control arrangements are established and implemented, and facilitating the execution and management of the health response to incidents and emergencies. This requires active participation in managing the response to incidents and emergencies. (It is important to note that not all RHEPAs have an on-call responsibility for major incidents.)

- Playing an active part in the design, establishment and efficient operation of any regional crisis management centre or control room.

- Ensuring that robust arrangements exist for dealing with CBRN incidents and establishing Joint Health Advisory Cells (JHAC).

- Maintaining and reviewing emergency plans and facilitating training to conform with Department of Health guidance and the principles of integrated emergency management.

- Coordinating and participating in the preparation, umpiring and evaluation of training and exercises and the debriefing of incidents. Furthermore, analysing lessons identified to inform and amend national policy and guidance, and implementing best practice at all levels.

9.7 Joint Health Advisory Cell

The Joint Health Advisory Cell (JHAC) is a group of 'health' experts that can be activated by the Police Incident Commander in the event of a chemical, biological, radiological or nuclear (CBRN) incident. The JHAC comprises of a range of highly specialised people from various organisations, e.g. the Environment Agency, water companies, the military and emergency services, and includes toxicologists, microbiologists, epidemiologists and media officers. The role and responsibilities of the JHAC include:

- advising the Police Incident Commander, other emergency services, partner agencies and incident control teams on immediate actions required to protect themselves, health, the environment, and the consequences of any actions they are considering

- leading on public health and environmental aspects of media and public information in conjunction with emergency services

- continually assessing the situation and highlighting public health issues to the police, military and other responders as the issues emerge

- contributing to the risk assessment and providing advice in planning tactical operations by the police

- determining the population at risk

- making recommendations on food and water consumption and advising on remediation actions
- providing rapid advice on the need to shelter, evacuate or contain and quarantine
- assessing whether the situation has a possible deliberate element
- maintaining public confidence in the response to the incident.

9.8 Summary

This chapter has provided an overview of the roles and responsibilities of health organisations that exist at local, sector/county, regional and national level. As such, the roles of the Department of Health, the NHS and the Health Protection Agency have been discussed. The functions of the regional HEPAs and the JHAC have also been explored.

9.9 Notes

1. Section 9.2 is reproduced with the kind permission of the Department of Health.

10

Chemical, Biological, Radiological and Nuclear Incidents

Virginia Murray, Sarah Norman, Dilys Morgan, Jill Meara and Jim Stuart-Black

10.1 Introduction

Chemical, biological, radiological or nuclear (CBRN) plans and arrangements are not designed to be activated solely in response to a deliberate release incident: they can and should be utilised for any incident that involves chemical, biological, radiological or nuclear agents or materials. The term 'deliberate release' refers to any intentional spread of a CBRN agent, such as might occur in a bioterrorist incident. A release may be **overt**, i.e. clearly identifiable; there may have been a prior warning, or the release may be apparent, either due to the use of an explosive device or because a suspicious substance is obviously visible. Alternatively, a release may be **covert**, with a concealed release of a biological or chemical agent. In these circumstances, the release will not become apparent until the first symptomatic cases arise.

Emergency planning for these types of incidents is particularly associated with special detailed plans that require exercising and regular reviewing to develop the best available approach for managing the response to CBRN incidents. Guidance is available – readers should refer to the HPA (2005) publication by Heptonstall and Gent, *CBRN Incidents: Clinical Management and Health Protection*, in addition to a number of key websites which are provided in the annexes. This chapter includes sections on the following:

- an explanation of CBRN incidents with brief examples
- key information that should be included in a Trust's CBRN plan
- an explanation of how to identify CBRN incidents using 'Step 123' and advice on dealing with cases of unusual illness
- a brief explanation of decontamination and personal protective equipment (PPE)
- a brief outline of sampling needs and toxiboxes
- discussion of the UK Reserve National Stock for Major Incidents ('pods')
- an overview of sheltering, evacuation and countermeasures
- suggestions on documentation.

10.2 Chemical incidents

Many chemical incidents occur every year. The Health Protection Agency's Division of Chemical Hazards and Poisons (CHAPs) records over 1,000 incidents a year in England and Wales. As a result, the National Health Service (NHS) and other emergency services respond to chemical events fairly frequently (refer to Box 10.1). Chemical weapons were used extensively over the last century in numerous wars. However, not until the chemical terrorist attacks occurred in Japan in 1994 and 1995 (refer to Box 10.2) did the eyes of the world open to the chaos that could occur during a deliberate release of chemical agents. These incidents were the first reported use of nerve agents on civilians by a terrorist group. In both incidents the nerve agent sarin was used and highly populated areas were targeted.

Box 10.1 A small hazardous materials incident, October 2000 (Harrison et al. 2002)

A man collapsed [while] cleaning out an 'empty' trichloroethylene tank. Colleagues found him, removed him from exposure, called an ambulance and started resuscitation. Within 10 minutes the ambulance arrived with two paramedics who continued resuscitation. Medical assistance was requested and a doctor, another paramedic and [an] ambulance arrived within the next 15 minutes. During transfer to A&E advice was sought via Ambulance Control when chemical burns were noted on the patient's body. Further occupational health assessment was recommended for all paramedics, emergency scene doctor, A&E staff and other medical and nursing staff. A mobile decontamination unit was set up at the scene with decontamination, health checks and biological sampling offered. Those assessed included a fellow worker, other workers on the industrial estate, police, Fire Brigade and a passer-by. Nine in all were found to be positive to trichloroethylene, receiving secondary contamination and suffering poisoning.

Key considerations

- Limiting exposure to chemicals by decontamination is the most effective way of minimising harm to casualties: make sure your decontamination units and personal protective clothing are available, and that relevant staff are trained in their use. Remember to secure the Trust as soon as possible by shutting and locking external doors to prevent contamination of your Trust's buildings.

- Chemical incidents require rapid hazard and risk assessment: make sure systems for communication will inform all professionals within and where appropriate without your Trust to facilitate rapid response.

- Liaise with relevant people, e.g. Ambulance Trusts, Acute Hospital Trusts, consultants in communicable disease control, public health, Chemical Hazards and Poisons (CHAPs) Division, Health Protection Agency, environmental health officers and local authorities, and the Environment Agency.

- Make sure systems for biological and environmental sampling, treatment, and occupational assessment for response and recovery are in place to support an incident.

- Review all chemical incidents identified in your Trust, identify lessons to be learned, and share this information to improve response in future by using these lessons for exercises and reviewing plans.

Box 10.2 Tokyo, 20 March 1995

Sarin was released in the Tokyo underground during rush hour, from five devices placed on three subway lines. Twelve people died, 5,510 sought medical attention in 278 hospitals and clinics, 688 victims were transported to hospitals by ambulance and >4,000 casualties reached hospitals either on foot or by private transport (Okumura et al. 1998). About 25% (approximately 1,000 people) who reached medical facilities required hospitalisation. Of the 1,364 emergency personnel who were at the incident, 135 (9.9%) showed acute symptoms and received medical treatment (Wheeler 1999).

A short summary of some of the deliberate release chemical agents, speed of onset, main features and need for decontamination and treatment is given in Table 10.1. Presentation will depend on how the chemical exposure occurs, i.e. which route of exposure for how long a period. Individual susceptibility varies among the very young, very old and those who are pregnant, with those with pre-existing disease being potentially at greater risk.

Table 10.1 Summary of some of the potential deliberate release chemical agents

Chemical	Speed of onset	Main feature	Decontamination and treatment
Nerve agents e.g. Sarin, tabun, Cyclosarin, soman, VX	Immediate	Myosis (small pupils), bradycardia (slow heart rate), salivation, rhinorrhoea (runny nose), lacrimation, sweating, convulsions	• Decontamination for any exposure • Antidotes: atropine, pralidoxime, diazepam • Oxygen, symptomatic and supportive
Hydrogen cyanide by inhalation	Immediate	Headache, dizziness, vomiting, anxiety, ataxia (difficulty in movement), confusion, hyperventilation, convulsions, dyspnoea (difficulty in breathing), collapse	• Decontamination for skin contamination • Oxygen, symptomatic and supportive • Antidote: dicobalt edentate
Chlorine	Rapid	Coughing, choking, vomiting, difficulty in breathing, eye and skin irritation	• Decontamination for skin contamination • Oxygen, symptomatic and supportive
Phosgene	Rapid or delayed effects possible	Eye irritation, coughing, difficulty in breathing – latent phase – oedema phase	• Decontamination for skin contamination • Oxygen, symptomatic and supportive
Cyanide salts by ingestion	Ingestion 30–60 minutes	Headache, dizziness, vomiting, anxiety, ataxia, confusion, hyperventilation, dyspnoea (difficulty in breathing), collapse	• Oxygen, symptomatic and supportive • Antidote: dicobalt edentate
Mustard	Delayed for 2–6 hours	Nausea, vomiting, headache, erythema (redness of skin), eye, skin and respiratory tract irritation, blistering and pain	• Decontamination for any exposure • Oxygen, symptomatic and supportive and pain relief
Ricin	Delayed for approximately 6 hours	Flu-like symptoms, fever, leucocytosis (raised white cell count), multi-organ failure	• Decontamination for skin contamination • Oxygen if inhaled, symptomatic and supportive

10.3 Biological incidents

The history of the use of biological weapons is a long one, going back to the siege of Kaffa in the 14th century, when the attacking Tartar army hurled bodies of plague victims into the city, up to anthrax in letters posted in the US in 2001 (refer to Box 10.3). Defectors report that the former Soviet Union had an extensive biological weapons programme employing over 60,000 people and producing many tons of biological weapons, most of which remain unaccounted for (Alibek and Handelman 2000). Large-scale production of such agents may not be necessary to produce a significant outbreak, and most of the agents classified by Centers for Disease Control and Prevention (CDC)(USA) as posing the highest risk to national security are endemic in many parts of the world (Box 10.4). Although it would therefore be relatively easy for an informed person with access to these agents to be able to grow them in relatively simple conditions, it is more difficult to devise an efficient way of disseminating the agent. However, even a few cases of infection from a biological agent would cause widespread disruption.

Box 10.3 Anthrax in the US, 2001 (Jernigan et al. 2002)

In October 2001, just after the attacks on the World Trade Centre and Pentagon, a case of inhalation anthrax was identified in a man working at a media company in Florida. A national investigation was initiated to find other cases and identify the cause. Over the next six weeks, 22 cases of anthrax – 11 inhalation [cases], of whom five died, and 11 cutaneous (skin) cases – were identified. Twenty of these [individuals] were either mail handlers or [were] exposed at work where contaminated mail was processed or received, and two had no known exposure. Four envelopes containing anthrax powder were found: two had been posted to media personnel in New York City and two to senators, both of whom were in Washington. Extensive contamination of the mail processing centres led to their closure, and decontamination proved very difficult. There was widespread panic throughout the US and this quickly spread around the world, despite the fact there were no cases outside the US. An estimated 32,000 people received antibiotic prophylaxis. Despite intensive investigations, the perpetrator has not been charged.

Key considerations

- An overt release of a biological agent would need urgent public health action in addition to emergency services response, with facilities for identifying those exposed, decontamination, and providing chemoprophylaxis and information sheets. Plans should be in place for dealing with an overt release of a biological agent. These plans should be brought to the attention of staff and integrated into other major incident plans.

- Hold exercises to try out the plans. This will help identify gaps or logistical problems.

- Because there is an incubation period between exposure and development of symptoms, the release of a biological agent may not be apparent until people become ill. Patients may present in a variety of settings, and identification of the first cases may be difficult. The identification of an overt release would therefore rely on the vigilance of health-care workers and other frontline staff, and on the recognition of unusual clusters or manifestations of disease. Staff also need to be aware of who they should contact if they suspect something unusual is occurring.

- Not all deliberate releases are done with exotic pathogens: relatively common infections may be used – another reason for frontline staff to remain alert to the possibility of a deliberate release.

- If a biological release is suspected or confirmed, there needs to be increased surveillance to detect possible cases by informing health workers, along with consistent information for the general public.

Box 10.4 Salmonella in Oregon, 1984 (Torok et al. 1997)

In 1984, there was an outbreak of gastroenteritis among individuals who had eaten at salad bars in a town in Oregon, United States. A total of 751 people were affected and Salmonella typhimurium was found to be the cause of the outbreak. Although there was a close association between eating at the salad bars and being ill, the source of the infection was not identified. More than a year later it was discovered that the Rajneeshee cult had deliberately contaminated food items in the salad bars in order to influence local elections in their favour. They were found in possession of the same strain of salmonella that had caused the outbreak. They had obtained this from a commercial medical supply company.

A summary of some of the agents, their presenting features and prophylaxis or treatment is given in Table 10.2. Presentation of most of the agents depends on how the infection was disseminated and thus acquired, e.g. whether the organism was inhaled or ingested, or if it entered through abrasion of the skin. The onset of symptoms is also related to the infecting dose.

Table 10.2 Summary of some of the potential deliberate release biological agents

Agent	Presenting features	Prophylaxis or treatment
Anthrax Incubation period 1–7 days (but spores can remain dormant in lungs for many weeks)	Inhalational: Non-specific flu-like illness with cough followed 2–4 days later by severe respiratory infection. Rapid onset. Widened mediastinum on chest X-ray. Cutaneous: Raised itchy inflamed pimple which over 2–6 days progresses to a papule then a vesicle (blister) surrounded by extensive painless oedema (swelling), culminating classically in a black ulcer. Gastrointestinal: Severe abdominal pain, nausea, vomiting, watery/bloody diarrhoea. Note: may also present as bacteraemia/meningitis.	Ciprofloxacin or doxycline
Plague Incubation period 1–4 days	Pneumonic: Intense headache, malaise, fever, vomiting, prostration, cough and breathlessness, watery blood-stained sputum, sever respiratory infection. Multilobar consolidation/bronchopneumonia on chest X-ray. Patient infectious. Bubonic: Swollen, painful, tender lymph nodes with associated oedema and redness. Note: may also present in septicaemic/meningitic/pharyngeal forms.	Ciprofloxacin or doxycline
Smallpox Incubation period 7–17 days	Fever, severe prostration, severe headache, 2–3 days later a maculopapular rash mainly on the face/extremities. This progresses over 5–6 days to classical pus-filled blisters. Rash may be haemorrhagic or flat. Patient is infectious.	Vaccination if within 4 days of exposure

Table 10.2 *continued*

Agent	Presenting features	Prophylaxis or treatment
Botulinum toxin Incubation period 1 hour–8 days	Acute onset of bilateral cranial nerve involvement. Descending weakness or paralysis, which may extend to complete flaccid paralysis. The patient remains alert with no loss of sensation and no fever.	Botulinum antitoxin if symptoms
Tularaemia Incubation period 1–21 days	Many different forms depending on route of infection: Pneumonic (acute flu-like +/- clinical pneumonitis/pneumonia) Ulceroglandular (local itchy papule develops into pus-filled blister and then into ulcer plus lymph node enlargement) Typhoidal (flu-like plus diarrhoea and vomiting) Oculoglandular (corneal ulceration plus lymph node enlargement) plus septicaemic or pharyngeal forms.	Ciprofloxacin or doxycline
Viral haemorrhagic fever Incubation period 2–21 days	Variety of clinical presentations depending on virus. Symptoms include fever, headache, muscle and joint pains and rash, followed by bleeding and shock. Patient is infectious.	Ribavirin may be useful for some viruses

10.4 Radiological and nuclear incidents

On a worldwide basis, both nuclear and radiological accidents and incidents are relatively infrequent when compared with events involving other potentially hazardous materials such as chemicals. In the UK, nuclear and radiological accidents are rare, the only major nuclear accident having occurred at Windscale, Cumbria, in 1957. Consequently, virtually no NHS personnel are likely to be experienced at dealing with the potential outcomes of nuclear accidents. Indeed, the public health consequences, even for a significant accident such as those on which nuclear site emergency plans are based, are likely to be small in terms of radiation-induced health effects. Similarly, for radiological accidents, whilst small-scale incidents and accidents have occurred in the UK over recent years, only a very limited number of NHS personnel are likely to have been involved in the response.

Box 10.5 The Chernobyl accident, 1986 (McColl and Prosser 2002)

The Chernobyl nuclear power station is situated approximately 100 km north of Kiev in Ukraine, close to the town of Pripyat. On 26 April 1986 tests were being carried out on one of the reactors, which led to an explosion that partially removed the reactor core lid, exposing the burning core and releasing radionuclides to the atmosphere. The release continued for at least 10 days. The extent and complexity of the radiological impact of the accident are not easy to summarise. Over 200 on-site workers developed acute radiation syndrome of varying severity. The resulting doses, some up to 16 Gy, were principally from external beta and gamma radiation. No member of the public was diagnosed as exhibiting acute radiation syndrome but over 135,000 people were evacuated and an exclusion zone of 30 km was established around the site. There have been approximately 1,800 childhood thyroid cancers observed to date but no other adverse health effects have been identified, contrary to current public perception.

Concerns regarding the potential malicious use of CBRN materials have increased following the heightened awareness of international terrorism post 11 September 2001. A variety of potential scenarios can be postulated involving either the deliberate release or emplacement of a radiological or nuclear source. In addition, public fears of all things radioactive, and the perceived complexity in understanding radiation concepts (see Table 10.3), have exacerbated potential fears. To date no known CBRN incidents involving radioactive or nuclear materials have been perpetrated in the UK, which is why much of the planning and preparation for responding to incidents involving these materials is based upon knowledge gained from exposure to radiation and radioactive materials in accident situations (see Boxes 10.5 and 10.6).

Table 10.3 Radiation: concepts and quantities

Radiation term	Explanation
Absorbed dose	Quantity of energy of ionising radiation imparted to a mass of tissue. Unit: gray (Gy).
Activity	Describes the quantity of radioactive material present. Unit: becquerel (Bq). Becquerels are not measures of radiation dose.
Decay	The decrease in activity of a radioactive substance with time. The rate of decay is dependent upon the radionuclide's half-life.
Half-life	The time taken for the activity to decay to half the original quantity ($t\frac{1}{2}$).
Radiation	The process of emitting energy as waves or particles. Frequently used to mean ionising radiation, i.e. radiation that causes ionisation in matter. Examples include alpha particles, beta particles, gamma rays, X-rays and neutrons.
Radionuclide	An unstable nuclide that emits ionising radiation.
Sievert (Sv)	A measure of radiation dose, i.e. the effective dose which takes account of the type of radiation and accounting for the effect on all of the organs in the body. Symbol: Sv. Smaller units are often used, e.g. millisieverts (mSv) – one thousandth of a sievert – or microsievert (μSv) – one millionth of a sievert.

Key considerations

- Radiation cannot be sensed by humans. Exposure to a radioactive source may not be immediately apparent unless large doses of radiation have been received.

- Exposure to radiation can produce one or more of the following effects: deterministic effects at high doses of radiation, stochastic effects at low doses, and psychological effects even where little or no radiation exposure has occurred.

- People can be exposed by various routes: inhalation of radioactive particles; ingestion of contaminated food or water; exposure from contamination of skin or clothes; and external exposure to a nearby radioactive source, contaminated area or object. Exposure can be limited by a number of methods depending upon the circumstances. These countermeasures can include sheltering, evacuation, decontamination, restriction of food and water, and stable iodine administration (the latter being effective to limit exposure from inhalation of radioactive iodine only; this is largely relevant to releases from operating nuclear reactors).

- The exposed population may fall into one of three categories:
  - irradiated (casualties who have received a large dose of radiation but who have no radioactivity on them)
  - contaminated (those who still have radioactivity on or in them)
  - irradiated and contaminated.

- Procedures should be in place for ensuring that monitoring of members of the public can take place if needed. This may need to include the capacity to conduct large-scale reassurance monitoring. Priority will be given to those members of the public at most risk, i.e. those exposed to the greatest levels of radiation dose. Other follow-up actions might be required, such as bioassay and assessment of any longer term risks.

- Decontamination is not an automatic or inevitable response to a CBRN incident involving nuclear or radioactive materials. The need for decontamination is dependent on the type and scale of the incident.

- Effective communication with the public and media is likely to be critical in the event of any incident that involves radiation or radioactive materials, even where the level of radiation dose and risk to public health exposure are low.

Box 10.6 Gioânia, Brazil, 1987 (International Atomic Energy Agency 1988)

Following the break up in 1985 of a medical partnership in a clinic in Gioânia, Brazil, a teletherapy unit containing a 50.9 TBq caesium-137 source was abandoned in the clinic's former premises, which were partly demolished. Some two years later, in September 1987, the source was removed from its protective housing by local people who had no knowledge of what it was and were simply after its scrap metal value. The source was in the form of a highly soluble caesium chloride salt, compacted to form a coherent mass within a doubly sealed stainless steel encapsulation. The source was subsequently ruptured and the radioactive caesium (a few hundred grams) was widely dispersed in the city. Many people incurred large doses due to both external and internal exposure, the symptoms of which were initially diagnosed as food poisoning. Four of these died and 28 suffered radiation burns. The extent and degree of contamination were such that seven residences and various associated buildings had to be demolished and topsoil had to be removed from a significant area. The decontamination of the environment took about six months to complete and generated some 3500m^3 of radioactive waste.

Some examples of potentially significant radionuclides, their main features and possible actions that could be taken to reduce/limit the radiation dose are given in Table 10.4. It must be stressed that the potential actions provided as examples are dependent upon a number of factors, including the scale and nature of the accident, rather than being critically dependent upon the radionuclide involved. It should also be noted that in medical or industrial uses of radioactive materials, generally sources contain only one radionuclide, rarely two. This contrasts sharply with the nuclear industry where a cocktail of radionuclides is present.

10.5 What's in a CBRN plan?

All Trusts must have subject-specific plans for CBRN incidents, which are kept in the annexes of the Trust's major incident plan. There is also a requirement to have a subject-specific plan for mass casualty incidents involving the management of large numbers of casualties. The management of CBRN incidents involves a multi-agency response (the roles and responsibilities of partner agencies are described in Chapter 8). The Trust must strive towards joint working with partner agencies to ensure a coordinated and integrated response to such incidents.

Table 10.4 Examples of potentially significant radionuclides

Radionuclide	Main features	Early actions to reduce or limit radiation exposure (NB critically dependent on scale and nature of accident)
Cobalt–60 Co-60	β/γ emitter t½ = 5.3 years Radiation sources in medicine and industry. Present in the nuclear fuel cycle.	Establishment of a cordon Sheltering Evacuation Decontamination
Strontium–90 Sr-90	β emitter t½ = 29.1 years Radiation sources in medicine and industry. Present in the nuclear fuel cycle.	Establishment of a cordon Sheltering Evacuation Decontamination
Iodine–131 I-131	β/γ emitter t½ = 8.0 days Radiation sources in medicine and industry. Present in the nuclear fuel cycle.	Establishment of a cordon Sheltering Evacuation Decontamination Administration of stable iodine
Caesium–137 Cs-137	β/γ emitter t½ = 30.0 years Radiation sources in medicine and industry. Present in the nuclear fuel cycle.	Establishment of a cordon Sheltering Evacuation Decontamination
Iridium–192 Ir-192	β/γ emitter t½ = 73.8 days Radiation sources in medicine and industry.	Establishment of a cordon Sheltering Evacuation Decontamination
Plutonium–239 Pu-239	α emitter t½ = 2.4 x 10⁴ years Present in nuclear weapons and the nuclear fuel cycle.	Establishment of a cordon Sheltering Evacuation Decontamination
Americium–241 Am-241	α emitter t½ = 432.7 years Radiation sources in industry. Present in nuclear weapons and the nuclear fuel cycle.	Establishment of a cordon Sheltering Evacuation Decontamination

Chemical plans could include:

- background/introduction
- risk assessment
- pre-hospital response (brief)
- principles of managing a chemical incident
- types of incident and notification
- large-scale incidents
- containment

- activation of the chemical incident plan
- preparation
- decontamination process:
  - wet decontamination – rinse, scrub, rinse
  - dry decontamination
  - disposal
  - treatment
  - patient clothing and possessions
  - sampling
  - debriefing.

(Adapted from St Bartholomew's and the Royal London Trust 2003)

Biological plans could include:

- background/introduction
- risk assessment
- pre-hospital response (brief)
- principles of managing a biological incident
- types of incident and notification
- large-scale incidents
- containment
- activation of biological incident plan:
  - preparation and infection control
  - decontamination of persons exposed
  - isolation of patients
  - cleaning disinfection and waste
  - prophylactic treatment for persons exposed
  - contacts of cases
- debriefing.

Radiological and nuclear plans could include:

- introduction
- classification of casualties:
  - external exposure
  - external contamination
  - internal contamination
- alert procedure
- the roles of the radiation protection adviser or deputy
- equipment for radiation incidents to be kept in the A&E department
- monitoring equipment kept by clinical physics
- preparation for casualties

- casualty decontamination:
  - general principles
  - casualty reception
  - decontamination team rules
  - decontamination procedure
  - treatment of casualties with external exposure
  - treatment of external contamination
  - treatment of internal contamination
- disposal of bodies
- stand-down procedure
- debriefing.

(Adapted from St Bartholomew's and the Royal London Trust 2003)

10.6 Mass casualty incidents

The term Mass Casualty denotes a major incident of catastrophic proportions. Because of its extreme scale and/or complexity, such an incident would actually or potentially overwhelm and incapacitate normal services and special arrangements for responding to Major Incidents (Bailey 2003).

The NHS must make suitable preparations to meet such an eventuality. Each Trust should include a subject-specific plan on mass casualties in its major incident plan. Trusts should consider the following planning principles and assumptions in a mass casualty incident:

- the NHS in the affected locality will be unable to function normally and may not be able to function at all
- the command, control and coordination structure may change to accommodate the management of such an incident
- normal standards of practice for clinical and support services may be unachievable
- emergency measures may be required to address health and safety issues in such an incident
- the aim will be to do the best possible for the greatest numbers with the available resources
- the normal infrastructure and essential support services necessary to function as normal will be unavailable or seriously impaired
- priority will be delivering an emergency service while planning for recovery of normal services.

Trusts should consider including the following in their mass casualty incident plans:

- definition of mass casualty incident
- Trust response
- clinical care
- capacity escalation
- command and control mechanisms
- debriefing.

10.7 Identifying a CBRN incident

The early identification of the type of incident (i.e. CBRN, conventional terrorism or other) will ensure a proportional and appropriate level of response from both the health organisations and the wider emergency planning community. Furthermore, health stakeholders need to be aware of the legal requirement identified in the Civil Contingencies Act for all Category 1 responders to 'maintain arrangements to warn the public, and to provide information and advice to the public if an emergency is likely to occur or has occurred.'

Accurate incident identification (type) will ensure effective resource management, particularly in the event of a hoax incident; furthermore, it will ensure that health organisations do not unnecessarily alarm the public, in accordance with the Civil Contingencies Act 2004.

Intelligence to warn of an overt event may be available. However, the need to identify an unexpected event (be it overt or covert) may be helped by including in planning and training programmes information such as STEP 123 or dealing with cases of unusual illness.

10.7.1 STEP 123

The Safety Triggers for Emergency Personnel (STEP 123) system was developed by London's blue light services as a simple scene assessment tool for use by all staff (Waspe 2003). The origin of STEP 123 lies within NATO (North Atlantic Treaty Organisation) procedures. As a system, it was easily transferred to civilian use and has become an integral part of the emergency services' response. STEP 123 is primarily used by those staff who are likely to be the first to arrive at the scene of an incident but have not received specialised training in CBRN or hazardous materials (HAZMAT) incident management. The STEP 123 protocol is used only when the cause of a collapse(s) is unknown, and when applied it will activate the necessary specialist response from all of the agencies tasked to deal with HAZMAT or CBRN incidents (refer to Table 10.5).

Table 10.5 STEP 123

STEP 1	ONE casualty	Approach using normal procedures
STEP 2	TWO casualties	Approach with caution, consider all options, report on arrival and update control
STEP 3	THREE casualties OR more	Do not approach the scene
		Withdraw
		Contain
		Report
		Isolate yourself
		Send for specialist help

10.7.2 Dealing with cases of unusual illness

Guidelines for dealing with cases of unusual illness appear on the Public Health Laboratory Service (PHLS) website (www.hpa.org.uk) and are summarised here. The critical factors in responding to unusual outbreaks or incidents are:

- maintaining a high level of awareness
- attending to the issues of patient decontamination, containment and staff safety when cases occur

- early expert clinical assessment of patients to consider the most likely cause before epidemiological and tests results become available, and the institution of rapid relevant investigations and management

- effective communication between different sectors of the health service and between the NHS and other relevant agencies

- effective coordination of the response by an overall incident management lead.

10.8 Decontamination

All those with a responsibility for decontamination should already hold/maintain specialist plans that have been developed in consultation with their Regional Health Emergency Planning Adviser (RHEPA) and other support agencies. What follows is a brief outline of some of the more salient points. It is important to note that the list is not exhaustive and serves merely as a guide. Further information is available from the Home Office (2004) publication, *The Decontamination of People Exposed to Chemical, Biological, Radiological or Nuclear (CBRN) Substances or Materials: Strategic National Guidance*, and the HPA (2005) publication by Heptonstall and Gent, *CBRN Incidents: Clinical Management and Health Protection*.

The decontamination process aims to remove clothing and skin contamination without endangering health-care workers. All those involved in the decontamination of people exposed to CBRN substances or materials must have a common set of principles, and they need to use common terminology and have a shared and agreed understanding of each others' roles and responsibilities. Once the decision to decontaminate has been made (dependent on the assessment of the incident by first responders), the principle is that all casualties (whether injured or not) who are suspected of being contaminated will receive decontamination at the scene. It is important for all Trusts (not just Acute Trusts) to be prepared for people who may self-refer, and who may not have been decontaminated at the scene.

If decontamination procedures are initiated, it is important to be aware of the roles of all organisations and agencies involved (refer to Chapter 8) and to know how systems have been developed to try and minimise harm (Figure 10.1). These are described as zones which can be defined as:

- The 'hot' zone: only the fire brigade or military in full personal protective equipment (PPE) may enter. The police may enter the hot zone (if in appropriate PPE) to identify secondary devices.

- The 'warm' zone: where clinical, emergency and mass types of decontamination are undertaken. (An **inner cordon** separates the hot and warm zones.)

- The 'cold' zone: for patient assessment and dispatch to medical care as required. (An **outer cordon** separates the warm and cold zones.)

10.8.1 'Clean' and 'dirty' zones

As part of all decontamination activities, it is essential to separate casualties awaiting decontamination in the contaminated area (or the 'dirty' zone) from those who have been decontaminated (in the 'clean' zone). In order to ensure that patient and staff safety can be maintained in the clean zone, it is vital that contaminated casualties do not cross from the dirty zone into the clean zone. Trusts should consider having large quantities of easily accessible tape to designate zones rapidly.

10.8.2 Personal protective equipment

In 2002, all Acute and Ambulance Trusts in England were issued with personal protective equipment (PPE) and portable decontamination units by the Department of Health, to increase the preparedness of the NHS to respond to the possibility of a small number of self-presenting casualties in Acute Trusts, and to allow Ambulance Trusts to treat a small number of contaminated casualties at the scene of a CBRN incident.

10.8.3 Decontamination

- The first objective is to remove the contaminated person from the area of greatest contamination (usually into open air and upwind of the incident).

- The careful removal of contaminated clothing will reduce the level of contamination and should, therefore, be a priority. Special care must be taken to ensure there is no spread of contamination from any clothing to exposed skin. Clothing should then be stored away from emergency services staff and other casualties, in labelled clear plastic bags and in a secure area, for evidence retrieval, decontamination if possible or destruction as appropriate.

- Types of decontamination:
    - **Clinical decontamination** is carried out by an Ambulance Trust, which can decontaminate both mobile and non-mobile casualties.
    - **Emergency decontamination** is carried out with the assistance of the Fire Service and may include low-pressure water spray from a fire hose, portable showers, and the use of large, purpose-built mobile units and fixed facilities away from the scene of the incident, or any other water source.
    - **Mass decontamination** is used for large numbers of people/casualties requiring decontamination and may include low-pressure water spray from a fire hose, portable showers, the use of large, purpose-built mobile units and fixed facilities away from the scene of the incident, or any other water source.

- Depending on the nature of the incident, an entrapped casualty may have to be partially decontaminated in situ.

- Casualties who have undergone decontamination will need further clinical assessment and may need further treatment.

- The deceased must be treated with respect and dignity. During the immediate response, unless they are presenting a hazard to the living, the deceased should where practicable be left in situ. Specialised body bags and other equipment may be necessary to minimise harm to others.

10.8.4 Training for CBRN incidents

In addition to the provision of appropriate equipment, there is also a requirement for training. Consequently, a nationally funded training standard, 'the structured approach to chemical casualties' (SACC), was commissioned by the Department of Health. This has been cascaded down to individual practitioners in all emergency departments in England. The aim of this half-day individual skills course is to ensure staff understand the use and limitations of the NHS-specified PPE, as well as the method and limitations of individual casualty decontamination, and the initial and further treatment of chemical casualties, particularly for those chemicals identified as likely to be used in a deliberate release scenario. The Trust key trainers now have responsibility to deliver the SACC course to all staff within their respective emergency departments who potentially have a role in the management of contaminated casualties. Training continues to be offered with regular refresher courses in each of the regions.

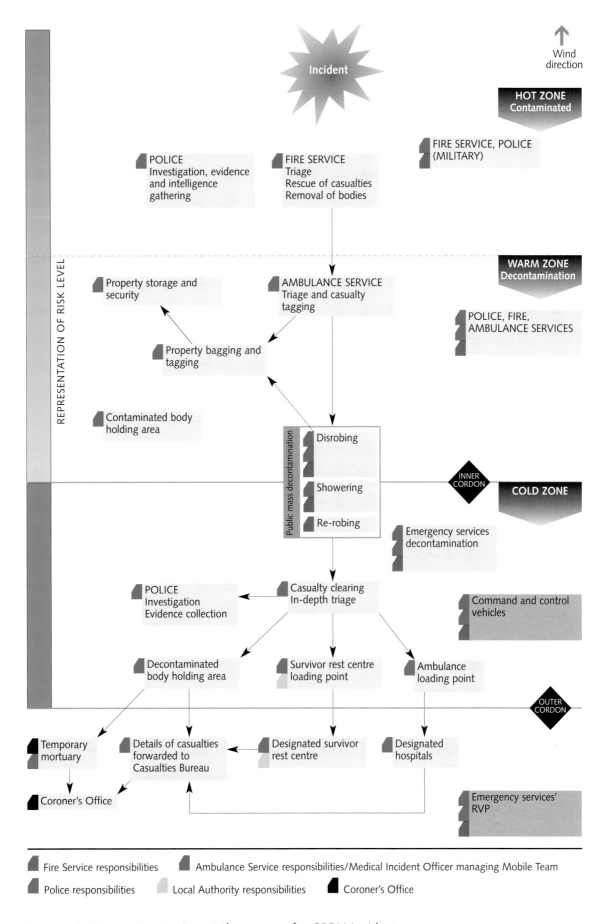

Figure 10.1 Decontamination at the scene of a CBRN incident

10.9 Sampling

Patients who have been exposed to CBRN substances may require urgent sampling. It is important that clinicians are aware of what equipment is necessary for these types of specialised tests. Examples include:

Chemical agents:

- Chemical 'blind screen'
  These blind screens have special kits – toxiboxes – with relevant instructions for adults and children, and should be available in A&E departments and Ambulance Trusts.

Biological agents:

- Microbiological 'blind screen'
- Respiratory tract samples
- Nose and throat swabs
- Pus and vesicle fluid or swab of local lesions if present
- Biopsy tissues
- Faeces/stools
- Other body fluids.

Further information on post-incident sampling can be found in the Department of Health (2000) publication, *Deliberate Release of Biological and Chemical Agents: Guidance to Help Plan the Health Service's Response* and the HPA (2005) publication by Heptonstall and Gent, *CBRN Incidents: Clinical Management and Health Protection.*

10.10 UK Reserve National Stock for Major Incidents ('pods')

These resources are intended to enhance the NHS' capacity and its ability to respond to major incidents, including mass casualty situations. They deal with the pre-distribution, mobilisation and delivery of the UK Reserve National Stock for Major Incidents, in the form of pre-packed 'pods' (containers). The pods are designed to enhance and support the capability of hospitals and Ambulance Services in providing airway management, administering antidotes, and clothing casualties when dealing with the consequences of CBRN or conventional incidents (Department of Health 2001). They include:

- equipment pods
- immediate drug kits
- nerve agent antidote pods
- dicobalt edetate pods
- modesty pods.

'Pod-holding' Ambulance Services may need to deliver pods to:

- receiving hospitals
- the scene of an incident
- emergency casualty treatment centres
- a holding point en route to one of the above locations.

In the event of an incident, non-pod-holding Ambulance Services should request delivery from the nearest appropriate pod-holding Ambulance Trust.

10.11 Sheltering, evacuation and countermeasures

The decision to shelter or evacuate in a conventional, accidental or deliberate release event is taken either with prior warning of an incident or as an incident is developing. In particular, it is essential that health stakeholders (via the Health Protection Agency) should be party to the decision-making process, and therefore they must not only collaborate closely with the emergency services in planning, but also participate in debriefing on incidents in order to develop good practice. In most cases the decision to evacuate will not be health led but will be taken by the emergency services. Although chief executives and other senior health managers are in charge of their health facilities, they need to heed the advice from the emergency services if sheltering or evacuation is recommended.

The Health Protection Agency will play a key role in providing public health advice about an incident that may result in advice to shelter or evacuate. NHS Direct (**telephone: 0845 4647**) can provide a vital nationwide link for medical advice before, during and following an incident involving sheltering or evacuation, and for the monitoring of possible cases.

10.11.1 Sheltering

Sheltering (refer to Box 10.7) is the action of seeking protection inside a building and preventing air from entering the building, e.g. if inside a hospital or medical clinic, this will mean closing all doors and windows, turning off any air conditioning and waiting for further instructions. A considerable degree of protection is afforded by sheltering in a house.

Effective communication systems must be in place to ensure that all those sheltered go outside to fresh air as soon as the hazard is safely past. If they stay sheltered too long, people may end up being exposed to a higher cumulative dose than they would receive if outside. Vulnerable groups may need assistance in their homes. Prompt medical attention may be needed after sheltering to triage those who may be at potential risk from hazards such as irritant gases.

Box 10.7 Effective sheltering

Go in, stay in, tune in

- Close windows and doors.
- Minimise draughts by sealing windows and doors with paper/tape or damp towels.
- Turn off central heating.
- Turn off mechanical ventilation including air conditioning (don't forget to give this advice to hospitals downwind of the plume).
- Go to an upper floor, and if possible to an interior room where ventilation is minimal.
- Avoid bathrooms and kitchens, which tend to have higher ventilation rates.
- Keep children and pets indoors.
- Breath through a wet cloth held over the face if the atmosphere inside becomes uncomfortable.
- Have access to a radio, and tune into the local radio station for further information and advice.

10.11.2 Evacuation

Evacuation is the action of leaving a building or location and seeking shelter in a safe location, e.g. a fire in a hospital may require an evacuation of patients either to another building, another hospital or alterative location. Evacuation should only be used as a measure of last resort when patients or staff are in serious danger. Specific instances could include:

Before an incident (precautionary)

- Risk of imminent explosion (e.g. defusing a Second World War bomb)
- Small leak likely to escalate sharply
- Threatened release of radioactive materials.

During an incident

- Spread of fire in a hospital or medical centre
- Continuing release of a chemical over a prolonged period of time.

After an incident

- Gross environmental contamination.

The decision to evacuate should always be taken in conjunction with the RHEPA and with health protection advice. The decision to evacuate may be affected by:

- the time required for deciding to evacuate by emergency services and health
- the time required to coordinate the notification to evacuate, e.g. door-to-door, via loudhailers, radio/TV networks, translation services
- the time of day
- the time necessary for the public to prepare to move – to collect clothes, medication, baby supplies, pets, cheque books, credit cards – and secure their homes
- the time taken to evacuate and the distance to a safe area, e.g. by car, walking, public transport, etc.
- the population characteristics of those to be evacuated, e.g. elderly, disabled.

10.11.3 Countermeasures

In a CBRN incident, it may be necessary to provide countermeasures to the affected community, such as immunisations, antibiotics, or other medication, to limit the effects of exposure to an agent. The Department of Health has developed 'Patient Group Directives' (PGDs), documents that make it legal for medicines to be given to groups of patients – for example, in a mass casualty situation – without individual prescriptions having to be written for each patient. They can also be used to empower staff other than doctors (for example, paramedics and nurses) legally to give the medicine in question.

It will be important, as part of the planning process, to develop arrangements for the distribution of countermeasures, including logistical arrangements, staffing and equipment needs and an appropriate location(s) for distribution. Further information about countermeasures and patient group directions is available online at www.dh.gov.uk

10.12 Documentation

As for any incident, the documentation of information is essential, and an accurate log must be maintained and accounted for. This must be done by all Trusts and any other health-care facility involved in the response. Health emergency planners will need to plan for the documentation needs of their service. An example of the process followed by public health is given in Box 10.8. The ongoing log of decision/actions/time is as important as the initial information and has legal ramifications for any subsequent public enquiries.

Box 10.8 Checklist of information to document

1. Who reported the outbreak/incident?
   - Name
   - Position
   - Organisation
   - Contact details.

2. How has the outbreak/incident come to light?

3. Where have cases occurred? Are there any common exposures recognised at this stage?

4. Over what time period have cases been detected?
   - What agencies are involved? Get contact details. Has a major incident been declared? Who else has been informed?
   - Is information available about the likely cause of the illnesses?
   - Is there evidence of deliberate action, e.g. threats received?

5. Who are the cases? Are they from a particular social group or setting?

6. How many cases are recognised at the moment?

7. Have the Health Protection Agency/Ambulance Service and local hospitals/GPs/NHS Direct been informed?

8. Where and how are the cases being managed?

9. Has decontamination of cases taken place? How?

10. Who else has possibly been exposed and therefore might be at risk of developing this illness? Has a list of them been made?

11. Are there any conditions occurring which might increase the risks to others, e.g. health-care workers exposed, ongoing incident, weather forecasts?

12. What is being done to prevent the development of new cases at the moment? For example:
   - protection of emergency and health-care staff
   - evacuation/sheltering
   - quarantine
   - prophylactic treatment.

10.13 Summary

This chapter has provided a brief explanation of the definitions of CBRN incidents along with a number of short examples. Key considerations have been provided to assist with the development of Trust CBRN plans, including advice on dealing with cases of unusual illnesses, decontamination procedures and PPE. The latter part of the chapter has provided information on toxiboxes, pods, shelter, evacuation, countermeasures and documentation.

11 Public Relations: the Added Value in an Emergency

Ann Fleming

11.1 Introduction

The best-laid plans can and will go wrong if you do not communicate them effectively, and although you may have organised all the other emergency planning operations to the *n*th degree, if the public information, media relations and internal communications planning is not on a par, then at best your handling of the entire crisis will be brought into question; at worst, your corporate reputation will take a knock from which it may never recover.

11.2 The public relations service

As soon as you take up your position as a health emergency planner, you need to make friends with your communications team and work closely with them. It should be a productive, mutually beneficial relationship.

Public relations teams, or communications teams, as they are often called, are responsible for making sure that the organisation's aims and objectives are understood, accepted and, if possible, favourably received by its publics; and that the organisation in turn understands the needs of the publics it serves or affects. They do this by strategically employing a range of promotional and communications skills, which can include media relations, editing and managing websites, writing and editing publications, developing digital and broadcast media channels, marketing, event organisation, public affairs, and media and customer service monitoring and analysis. This list is not exhaustive.

Public relations officers, like emergency planners, are skilled in seeing and anticipating all possible outcomes from what could be the most seemingly innocuous situation. They are horizon scanners and as such play an important role in your organisation's strategic decision making process. Therefore, it is important to include public relations activity in your risk assessments. Too often the service provided can be viewed as a purely technical one limited to drafting press statements and producing publications. If public relations is relegated to being an afterthought – if, for example, your meetings end with: 'Right, what should we put in the press release?' – you are misusing your public relations function, or you have not recruited practitioners at a sufficiently senior level to operate in the influential coalition where the service belongs. Public relations is a core function of the most successful companies and organisations and not a 'bolt-on' extra.

Your public relations team use their research and analysis skills on a daily basis to choose the most opportune moment actively to publicise a new campaign to best advantage or to organise a reactive response on a specific issue. In both cases they make sure that the messages are clear, credible, well timed and appropriately targeted for the intended audience. This can mean clarifying technical information for the lay reader or listener, or making sure that translations are available for minority communities.

Above all, public relations officers make sure that messages are consistent. This is vital if your organisation is to be perceived as an honest and authoritative source of information. The public may not like what you have to say, but if what you are saying to the media and in your public literature is the same as what you are saying to your staff and your stakeholders – and if this is supported by corporate behaviours – then you will maintain public and employee confidence. However, if the left arm does not seem to know what the right arm is doing, the media and the public will see a deliberate attempt to deceive; they will not see it as a temporary communications breakdown. The result is that all your future messages will go unheard, or certainly disbelieved.

The public relations unit is the organisation's eyes and ears: it acts as an early-warning system capable of telling which way the wind is blowing and of using this intelligence to maximise opportunities as well as to prepare for threats. In fact, in our defence of the corporate reputation, we risk being viewed as a Cassandra figure, but from your point of view, you have an ally whom, having prophesied doom, should be working alongside you to limit the potential damage.

11.3 Media relations preparations

You may have only just made your introductions to the public relations team and they might not yet have a written emergency procedure or plan for communications. However, they will have laid the important foundations for emergencies on their first day in post. The linchpin of crisis communications is a professional and mutually respectful relationship with the media. Undoubtedly, you can make and strengthen these relationships in a crisis. However, you will be on a much firmer footing if, prior to a crisis, you know someone's style and their approach to their work, their audience, their deadlines, the slant to their work and their chosen means of receiving information. This way you should be well on the way to becoming the 'trusted' authority.

The aim is that journalists, through repeated positive interactions with your organisation, recognise it as a reliable authority and one that gives timely and honest information in good times and bad. The professionalism of your public relations team on a day-to-day basis will single out your organisation as a truthful and authoritative source of information in a crisis. They know how to work with each medium; they know how to craft copy and tailor content for different editorial requirements; and they can empathise with different readerships, viewers and listeners.

However, this level of professionalism is not achieved by the public relations team alone: it is attained by a culture where the public relations department exerts influence. Here media awareness runs like a vein through every tier of the establishment, so that managers prioritise media enquiries and can alert the public relations team to good news stories and elephant traps.

A media-aware organisation knows that internal newsletters, documents and emails find their way to the press, whether covertly or via the freedom of information route. And it knows that news breaks at the click of the 'send' button and that journalists attend public meetings at the invitation of protagonists. It may not appreciate what eventually appears on the page or on screen, but it respects the fact that the media has a mandate to scrutinise rigorously the work of public bodies.

It is hard to fathom, but some organisations still underestimate the power, the immediacy and the breadth of the media. The rapid technological advancements in the digital age have given added meaning to the term 'mass media'. It has made us all potential reporters, whether by design – having our own blog site on the internet – or by circumstance, as in the case of a citizen reporter photographing and emailing the immediate aftermath of a crash or a terrorist bomb from a mobile phone. Traditional routes of promoting services, products and positions are being bypassed in favour of approaches once considered to be guerrilla tactics.

It is not logistically possible to feed or respond to all media opportunities or requests of this nature, but it is possible to mitigate for them. You do this by publicising your successes not only via the media but through internal communications with your workforce, through your external publications and events, and by keeping your web pages bang up to date with your company's ethos and its position on topical issues, summarised in plain language and a clean style.

We will look closer at media statements and media spokespeople in a crisis when we come to look at the joint communications strategy.

11.4 Media on side

Getting information out quickly and accurately in an emergency can save lives. This is why each region in England and Wales has a Regional Media Emergency Forum (RMEF). These were set up as a voluntary arrangement, bringing together senior media representatives and communications managers from Category 1 and 2 responder organisations in order to develop the best public information and news practice for emergencies.

Through the RMEFs, the media gain a better understanding of how the emergency response works and an insight into why there may be constraints in reporting. The communication managers advance their knowledge on what the media requires and the role that the media can play in warning and informing the public – a legal requirement for Category 1 and 2 responders under the Civil Contingencies Act. All in all the meetings are a vehicle for developing trust between the different agencies, which is essential if we are to work effectively together under pressure.

The Government News Network (GNN), the regional communications service for the government, acts as secretariat for the RMEFs, which are chaired in several areas by a representative from the British Broadcasting Corporation (BBC). The BBC, paid for by the public purse, takes its role as a public service broadcaster seriously, and has developed its 'Connecting in a Crisis' initiative to explain to the emergency planning community how to work effectively with the corporation to issue essential information to the public in times of crisis.

However, the BBC is by no means alone in believing it has such a duty. The RMEFs have media members from independent broadcasting organisations and the print media, who put their public information duties on an equal footing with that of the corporation.

The meetings afford an excellent opportunity to test media protocols, share good practice, look at technological innovations, and discuss joint working and communication networks. The feedback from short-lived, localised incidents, such as how to cater for satellite vans, press accreditation issues and business continuity for the media industry, is invaluable.

11.5 Internal communications

When we really want to know what is going on, when we think there is a further truth behind the headlines and the corporate speak, we want verification from the horse's mouth. That means we look for an organisation's employees. Knowing 'someone who works there' and listening to what they have to say complements the official line and is more compelling than any article or broadcast. This is just one of the reasons why it is vital that your workforce knows the details of the big issues facing the organisation, even if it will have very little impact on their own work in the short term. It does not give confidence to the public when employees tell them that the first they knew about it was in the press – although with advancements in technology, this is becoming more difficult to manage.

There will, of course, be employees who you will specifically need to inform. These are the staff operating the public helplines, or who are at the scene or treating the casualties. The information you give out to these people must be aligned and consistent with the messages you are giving out in public, or it will be seized upon by casualties, their families, the media and the public alike.

Some companies have taken the step of setting up secure web pages or intranet sites, which staff can access from home. Knowing whether you should or should not attempt to get into work following a major incident, and providing the latest information in briefings, allows employees to organise their working day and their personal lives. This sort of information helps create better ambassadors for the organisation.

Third party endorsement from an employee, a client or a stakeholder is powerful, which is why the technique is often used in advertising and highlighted by research. However, unplanned, informal endorsement by an employee is a potent force to be reckoned with.

This is why your public relations office should actively engage staff and issue as much information as you have to hand. If you do not have all the details to hand, tell them so and let them know when they will be fully briefed. If you do not provide information through recognised internal communications channels at the time you specified, then speculation through the grapevine will quickly fill the void you have left behind.

11.6 The emergency media and public information strategy

Your organisation's communications strategy for emergencies will not work if it is ratified by your senior management after one draft, only to remain on the shelf until disaster strikes. It must be shared and revisited and updated on a regular basis.

No organisation, and probably no sector (with the possible exception of the police), manages its crisis communications in isolation. This is why the joint communications strategy, containing media handling protocols, media centre operations, and joined-up messages and behaviours, can be a problematic document to prepare.

For health it means defining roles and communications channels, rotas and generic public health messages for every eventuality in the area. This means that Acute NHS Trusts, Primary Care Trusts, Regional Strategic Health Authorities, including the Regional Director of Public Health, the Health Protection Agency (HPA), NHS Direct, the Ambulance Service and private health trusts, all have to be factored into your plan, and together they must provide and agree roles and the content, language and tone of public health information, whether this is information to households following a chemical fire, infection control procedures, or when dealing with mass casualties.

The final joint communications strategy should set out a protocol for the handling of media and public information to be operated by all the agencies. It should specify and set up a mechanism to allow all relevant agencies to agree public information prior to its release. It should also emphasise the responsibility every agency has to share information with its partners. Each joint communications strategy is a very detailed document, which specifies roles and provides templates for statements and records; and therefore it is not beneficial to reproduce one here. However, any strategy will also state that only some sections will apply in any given situation.

The communications strategy should be ratified by all agencies, the communications leads of the Local Resilience Forums (LRFs) and members of the Regional Civil Contingencies Committees (RCCCs). It should be shared at the RMEF, so that the emergency services, regional government representatives and the media know who to contact and where to locate vital public health information.

Although the chain of command and control will be spelled out clearly in your local emergency planning procedures and more widely in the major incident plans, the communications strategy will focus on which organisation leads on media liaison. This is the tangible evidence to the public that this is the organisation with the key responsibility for managing the disaster. In the majority of incidents it will be the police who lead and manage the media operations, although occasionally this could fall to the Fire Service. This is why most Local Resilience Forums have a police lead on their communications group. In a major incident there will be a designated role for every public relations officer from every relevant Category 1 and 2 responder organisation, whether this is managing media accreditation for a media centre, media liaison, maintaining a media log and providing a media monitoring service, or briefing spokespeople and politicians.

The lead organisation for the media may not be the organisation that provides the expert spokesperson. Remember: all Category 1 and 2 responders have a responsibility to warn and inform, but not to alarm. In the event of a sustained crisis, such as pandemic influenza, the expert spokesperson may be a regional government representative, a health specialist or even an emergency planner!

11.7 Media training

If this is ringing alarm bells we should move on to media training. Your organisation will also need to anticipate different emergency scenarios in order to decide who it will field for media interviews. The public relations team can then organise robust media training for those individuals and also make sure that this training is repeated on a regular basis. The handling of the crisis and the reputation of your organisation are vested in the performance of your interviewee.

If your public relations team think that you are a likely candidate for interviews, then you should demand media training. It may be that you have had training some years ago and you think this will suffice. It will not. Time has moved on. Technically, it is now quite normal to have to give testing live interviews to a microscopic unmanned camera with no guidance on where your eyes should focus, no video link into a studio, and no relationship with your interrogator. Culturally, the nation now seeks to apportion blame and pursue recompense through the courts.

This chapter will not go through interview techniques. In a crisis you need practical instruction on how to prepare, perform and appear. The thought of media training can be daunting and you may feel that you are leaving yourself exposed in front of colleagues. Try to liberate yourself from such fears and demand the most vigorous training – you are expected to make mistakes: if you did not, you would be the trainer. Media training pays!

However, prior to training, an emergency planner or a chief executive can still plan for the killer questions such as: 'You tell us you have been planning for this, yet we are two days into this and the health service is in meltdown.' Remember that contrary to popular myth reporters do want to pass on important information for the public. Many of us perform well under pressure but fold under questions that begin: 'Tell me about . . .'

When it comes to applying this training in a live situation, your public relations officer will first of all assess the reporters' needs and the angle they intend to take. They want to make sure you are the most appropriate person to do the interview. They will also establish boundaries for the interview by letting reporters know beforehand what you are qualified to talk on and where they should seek out any extra information they require. The public relations office will state that the organisation is not going to speculate on unknowns or areas where they have no responsibility. If this is pursued during the interview it is entirely reasonable to repeat on air that you have said that you will not engage in conjecture.

Your public relations team should also organise media awareness training for all staff who, in their field of work, could find themselves on the front line in an emergency. The media will always want to talk to eyewitnesses or people dealing with the aftermath of an emergency. This is a legitimate request, and therefore if your organisation seems obstructive you risk being seen as guarded, therefore hiding something, or officious.

Neither of these achieves the desired image. So the aim, on one hand, is to prevent employees at the scene looking and behaving like rabbits caught in the headlights; on the other, it is to prevent overconfident individuals recasting themselves as the chief health official. Guidance on how to facilitate media needs politely, and how to retain the confidentiality of casualties and not issue any sensitive information, should all be included in the training.

If the emergency is going to be prolonged, and if there is a risk that public relations officers may be affected, which could happen in an influenza pandemic, then other employees may have to learn the basic technical public relations skills to achieve business continuity. This training could be provided in-house by the public relations manager and reinforced with short secondments to the team.

There is one more important aspect of media training for an emergency. Your public relations officers should be fully aware of and be able to apply legislation relevant to media handling in a disaster. This includes the Data Protection Act, Freedom of Information Act, the Human Rights Act and rules governing copyright and libel.

11.8 Reference material

Your own emergency communications plan and the joint media handling protocol should have an appendix with a list of designated media spokespeople for the organisation, their areas of expertise, and their contact details in and out of hours. The list should have more than one person in each area of expertise, to take into account annual leave commitments, for example, and to provide resilience if the emergency is a pandemic.

Public relations managers in the health sector should, in readiness for any emergency, have prepared emergency contacts lists with out-of-hours details for all key personnel in the organisation. This should include the executive team, administrators, customer service staff, relevant stakeholder personnel and of course media contacts. They should also have drawn up a press office rota for the emergency, which can be absorbed into an emergency press facility.

Together with you and other managers and clinicians, your public relations team will have prepared question and answer sheets, which can be used to form the basis of public information leaflets or as reactive responses to the media. These can be on anything from the symptoms of radiation poisoning to the trauma of a bomb attack or the symptoms caused by exposure to toxins from a chemical fire.

Generic public health messages and prepared statements should also be drafted in partnership to cover most health emergencies, and they should be agreed and signed off by stakeholder executive groups in your region. In nearly every emergency public health messages and media statements come from organisations on the ground, and it may be local practitioners in hospital or emergency services at the scene. However, in an emergency with nationwide implications, such as a flu pandemic, the media messages will be developed and issued by the government's News Co-ordination Centre (NCC), which feeds into the Cabinet Office Briefing Room (COBR).

The first media release issued in a crisis is often referred to as a holding statement; that is, a statement to acknowledge an exceptional incident pending more information. These statements do not have to be devoid of details. If the nature of the incident is known then you have your public health messages; if it is not, you can describe who is doing what, where and why, and say when further information will be available.

There must be a clear sign off procedure for media statements so that there are no surprises when the media pack descends and everyone is under pressure and in the limelight. This protocol can be developed beforehand but will need to be confirmed once RCCC and Gold command stand up.

Now is also the time to establish briefing mechanisms for spokespeople. Key messages that come from the relevant specialist units should, where possible, be seen in an emergency by a Director of Public Health or a Medical Director and go out in their name to the elected spokesperson and the public relations team. If these mechanisms are not in place, there is a danger of exposing senior officers and issuing conflicting information. This could endanger public health and damage your corporate reputation at the time of the emergency and later if there is a judicial review.

One particular emergency communications channel, the value of which cannot be overstated, is the website. An emergency communications plan should include a 24-hour web service so that the latest press statements, transcripts or recordings of media interviews – and the latest images – can go online immediately. This will help to satisfy regional and local media from other areas of the country, and the international media, leaving your media centre to cope with the reporters and camera crews who have arrived on your doorstep.

Public relations representatives from all relevant stakeholders should work together to develop communications action cards, which should be available for duty press officers to indicate who to contact in an emergency, and where to access statements to tailor to issue in the first hours of the plan.

11.9 Media and public information operations facility

Your public relations team will need the emergency planning officer's assistance to set up an emergency media centre. This needs to be as near as possible to the central operations room, so that the dedicated spokesperson, who will probably be sitting in Gold command or the RCCC, is never too far away from the centre. It must also be near the scene, because you want the media to use the facility. If it is an effort to get the centre, reporters and camera crews will be wary of missing photo and interview opportunities and may look elsewhere for information, some which may be inaccurate or pure speculation.

The centre will need an area for press conferences; an area separate from the press for briefing spokespeople and politicians; an area for the press to write and file copy; a reception area; an office for public relations officers to write statements; and a refreshments area, toilets and car parking facilities. The centre should be sited so that broadcast media can operate satellite vans in the facility.

You should equip the centre with power sockets, ISDN lines, satellite phones, mobile phones, telephone answering machines, two-way radios, computers with wireless connectivity, printers, fax machines, radios, televisions and recording equipment, software for uploading on to the internet, and logbooks as well as stationery. The public relations officers will need identification passes, press officer tabards and identification stickers for their vehicles.

It may be that you have a 'virtual' inter-agency press office, because a large media centre is not appropriate, even though you are in the midst of a crisis. An example of a prolonged calamity is pandemic influenza. The media will want to illustrate their reporting with localised human interest stories in hospitals, GP surgeries, the workplace and schools, and these bodies must be aware of this and plan accordingly. However, the media will want representation from the coordinating regional body. In this instance it may be wise to have a small press centre with an organised rota, and public relations officers across the region supporting the office in situ. This of course requires a strong agreed joint media strategy, and if the emergency is a pandemic, the overarching messages will come from national government.

11.10 Emergency exercises

You already know that you must regularly test your emergency response plans in exercises for both blue-light and rising-tide scenarios. Often exercises can rely heavily on media 'injects', which means that newspaper articles or television broadcasts are a device in the game to give players new information on the disaster.

In every exercise so far communications has been listed in the top three key issues in the concluding plenary session. Every public relations officer would be permanently ecstatic if such commitment to clear messages and serving the media were echoed in day-to-day practice. However, emergencies do raise awareness of these critical issues, so there is considerable room for optimism.

Exercises test so many critical areas of a plan, and it is not always possible to test media and public information communications because if you did, it would dominate proceedings. Exercises to test joint communications plans are invaluable, and this could be something you ask the Health Protection Agency to set up in conjunction with the Local Resilience Forum or RMEF. The lessons learned from such days can be shared with others outside the region and the participating agencies. However, one of the most valuable and necessary outcomes of these events is the strengthening of communications networks.

This may seem a contradiction, but many of the 'lessons learned' are not always learned. Revision is always useful. Revisit the report on the exercise or the last emergency that affected you and make sure that you have taken steps to address the actions. If the communications actions are not directly aimed at your own organisation, you should check that the public relations team in the relevant agency is aware of them. You cannot assume that they will have seen the report.

11.11 It's an emergency

As an emergency planner, you are one of the first people to hear of the emergency – you may even have been alerted by the public relations team. However, if this is not the case, make sure that one of your first calls is to alert the communications specialists. The initial stages of a disaster or emergency can be chaotic, and if the disaster happens out of hours, the media may well learn of the incident at the same time as you, if not before!

Quickly establish a single point of contact for the media (this may change as events unfold), which will issue operational media messages. Now is the time to issue your high-quality information and advice as soon as is possible, to avoid panic and unnecessary speculation.

11.12 The 'golden hour'

In emergency media relations, specialists refer to a 'golden hour', which in practice is often two hours. This is the critical time during which you must establish your organisation as a source of credible communication. You should issue your first public health messages within the first hour of the incident taking place.

You now need to establish where your key sources of information are and then make contact with them. These sources may be the police, the Acute Trust, the Radiological Protection Division of the HPA, or the Environment Agency.

The decision to activate the joint media plan will be made by the police after consultation with public relations personnel from the other affected organisations.

In the second hour you issue your now refined public health messages to the media and advise Gold command and the health advisory team, which will now have been stood up, of the health communications issues. This is when you will also need to agree lead health spokespeople from your trained pool.

This is an interesting conundrum. You have a major incident, and the media don't know about it yet. Who do you contact first? It is best to consider if you are warning or informing, or both. Do you need to influence behaviour? For example, if there is a major incident in a city centre on a Saturday evening, your main aim is to stop people coming into the centre. Your strongest media relationship may be your regional evening newspaper; they will want first-hand accounts and images, but they do not go to print until Monday. The demographics of the city centre probably indicate that you prioritise local and regional radio stations with a heavy music bias aimed at 16 to 30 year olds. This is also the group you will need to target with information sheets outside the cordon. Regional television is another important means of reaching the wider community.

In the golden hour your public relations officers will make a preliminary assessment of the extent of media interest and its expected duration. The public relations manager in charge has to manage the communications people in the area. This includes the forward planning for staff rotas, calling in GNN as support, if they are not automatically involved and if extra media handling is needed, and calling on support from colleagues outside the region. In addition to communications expertise technicians should be on hand to support the operation.

On-call public relations officers can be contacted and informed through the police and other agency text messaging alert systems. Once the joint media strategy has been activated, you must make sure that the mobile telephone numbers of each public relations officer are held by the emergency out-of-hours control room within their organisation. Now is the time to make sure that someone is managing the aligned internal and external communications plan, ensuring that the messages in both are consistent with what you are saying to the media.

Logbooks should record all the information released to the media, and there should be written transcripts of audio and video interviews. All press statements should be numbered, dated and timed, and the logbook should record the names and organisations of all the recipients. Pro forma can be organised beforehand to capture all these details.

If there is likely to be significant media demand then the decision will be taken to call in GNN press officers in addition to public relations staff from Category 1 and 2 responders. GNN is available 24 hours a day and is a regional government resource to boost and support the existing media operations where demand from the media outstrips the capacity to supply information. Emergency planning officers with an eye on budget control should be aware that GNN currently charge for any time subsequent to the first 24 hours of deployment.

However, you may still need to call in GNN for its role as part of the government information service. GNN provides national government departments and the Cabinet Office with media intelligence and handling advice. It is also responsible for organising all ministerial visits and will handle any media in Acute Trusts when politicians and VIPs visit to talk to victims. As previously stated, GNN coordinates the RMEFs and will cascade information to the BBC and other media so that the Civil Contingencies Act regulations to 'warn and inform' the public are met.

Designated public relations managers in health will put together briefings on the health response for all organisational tiers in health, and they will make sure that stakeholders within and outside the health sectors are briefed and that they in turn have mechanisms in place to cascade this information to all their employees. Press statements from health in emergencies should be approved by the health advisory team and seen by the lead police press officer in Gold command prior to release.

As involved as the public relations function is with the emergency, it will also be able to stand back from the emergency and with a cool eye scan the horizon for what is going to happen next. The conclusions must then be communicated through to Gold command before the public and media information for this next stage is prepared.

We have said before that the media operations centre for most emergencies will be managed by the police, and it is they who will manage media activity at the scene. Organisations need to be sensitive to the needs of casualties by protecting their confidentiality but also by respecting that casualties may have a very real need to speak to the media in order to make some sense of the situation in which they find themselves. When there are simply too many media representatives, or there is limited space or a sensitive interviewee, reporters and camera crews understand and are usually amenable to pooling resources.

11.13 Standing down the joint media communications strategy

The chair of Gold command and the senior public relations officer will make the decision to dissolve the joint media communications strategy arrangements. This will by no means mean the end of media interest; however, it does allow individual organisations to devise and issue their own media messages without referring to other stakeholders, although this may not be best practice. This is the time for organisations to promote their part in the emergency and describe the actions they are taking as a result. The public information and the press releases will be different to those issued by their partners in the event but they will not be contradictory.

The officers involved in the joint media strategy arrangements should meet after the dust has settled to discuss how the strategy worked, how it can be improved, the lessons learned, and in order to build on the newly strengthened relationships.

Media coverage about the incident, and about the media handling and the public information, can continue at intervals over several years. There may be a public inquiry, a judicial review, a plea for victims' compensation or simply a significant anniversary, and in these instances the public relations team can refer to the logbooks and share the line they intend to take with the other relevant organisations.

Finally, if you handled the media well, if you were open about mistakes made but you took actions in public view to make sure they did not happen again, and if your staff dealt sympathetically with the public and the media, then your corporate reputation should come out of the emergency not just unscathed but enhanced.

And, if you have not yet acquainted yourself fully with your public relations team, go and see them tomorrow, otherwise record it as a risk factor.

11.14 Golden rules for dealing with the media in a crisis

- Implement the joint media strategy and open the lines of communication as soon as possible.

- Refuse to speculate. At the beginning of a crisis reporters will all have the same information. By inviting the interviewee to speculate they are adding a unique selling point to their material and setting their paper or station apart from the rest.

- View the media as an asset. They are an invaluable means of getting out information quickly.

- Be proactive with bad news. If you issue a press statement announcing the news, you control the details, you will not be caught off guard by the journalist's questions, and you will demonstrate that you are open and honest in the most testing of times.

- Train customer service staff and switchboard operators to be vigilant. If a member of the public appears to be asking too many questions, they should take the caller's name and number and pass these details on to the public relations team.

- Treat all media even-handedly. If you show favouritism you will lose your position as an authoritative source of information among other reporters. However, if you need to prioritise, do so by order of deadlines.

- If the reporter is asking very general questions but you do not want to provide generalised replies, which could be misinterpreted, do ask them questions to pinpoint what angle they are taking and what it is they really want.

- Never say 'no comment'. If you do not have a mutually beneficial relationship with a reporter, do not provide information off the record. In fact, you should avoid talking off the record to all journalists. The quote may just be too irresistible for them not to use. National reporters will be much less likely to bother about protecting sources from regional or local organisations.

- Do express your sympathy or concern for casualties, victims and their families before you begin to outline your organisation's action plan, but be careful not to pre-empt police notification of next of kin in fatality situations.

- Do not implicate other people or organisations, no matter how unwittingly, in your dealings with the press.

- If you have made a mistake, say so and apologise openly, and then immediately say what you intend to do about it.

- If you are going to be interviewed, let stakeholders and colleagues know. They may already have provided the journalist with background information which you will not want to contradict.

- In the sound bite culture of the broadcast media, decide upon the key point you want to make, and plan how you intend to phrase it. If the interview goes beyond the expected sound bite and you have a terrier-like reporter trying to catch you out, simply repeat your point. If asked again, paraphrase your original point. If the interview is being recorded, it will most likely be edited down substantially prior to broadcast, and you don't want them to edit out your key message.

- Try to avoid jargon and acronyms. 'I am from the office of the RDPH and sit on the R triple C. I want to activate steps to optimise this opportunity …' Would YOU still be listening?

- Always keep a record of your responses and actions so you are not caught out later by reporters with a long memory or by the archives.

12

Organisational Debriefing and Reporting

Sarah Norman

12.1 Introduction

The National Audit Office (NAO)(2002) report stated that the:

> … Emergency Planning Co-ordination Unit [now known as the Emergency Preparedness Division] guidance requires a thorough debrief after major exercises and major incidents, so that lessons learned can be analysed and, if appropriate, incorporated into the Trust's plan. This should also assist in the sharing of good practice in handling major incidents, and reduce recurrences.

In addition:

> Post-event learning is an essential aspect of health emergency planning. Because major incidents occur on an infrequent basis, it is particularly important to document any lessons identified from managing incidents and to change current procedures and plans and provide reasons for any changes, so that they can be referred to in future incidents, which may not be managed by the same team. Any necessary organisational changes or amendments to emergency plans should be clearly detailed and a named person should be made responsible for ensuring that actions are carried out by a specified date. Many of the lessons identified in managing an incident have value for others working in the field. Wherever possible, incidents should be written up and published for the wider health community (Eagles et al. 2003).

This chapter will explore the post-incident activities that should be undertaken by the Trust, including:

- recovery activities, enabling a return to 'business as usual'
- support mechanisms for staff, and
- three types of organisational debriefing, which can be used to promote post-event learning:
  - the 'hot' debrief
  - the Trust debrief
  - the multi-agency debrief.

The chapter will also suggest a process of reporting and reviewing of plans and arrangements after the debriefing period has been completed.

12.2 Recovery activities for the Trust

Once the response phase has been completed, the responsibility for coordinating the multi-agency aspects of the recovery phase usually (but not always) moves from the Police Service to the local authority. Trusts will need to liaise closely with the local authority during recovery, to ensure health stakeholders are actively engaged as the focus of activity changes. It does need to be recognised that the recovery of your organisation and the community may last for a period of days, weeks, months, years or even decades. This circumstance may impact directly on your organisation's resources, including staff welfare, service provision and the relationship between the Trust and the community.

Following a major incident, the Trust may need to undertake a number of recovery activities, which may include (but may not be limited to) some or all of the following:

- physical reconstruction of facilities
- reviewing key priorities for service provision and restoration
- mid- to long-term community support and medical services
- long-term case management
- long-term public health issues
- financial implications, remunerations and commissioning agreements
- staffing and resources to address the new environment
- the socio-economic effect of the incident on staff and the public
- very important person (VIP) visits
- funerals, memorials and anniversaries
- staffing levels, welfare and resilience
- routine annual performance targets
- the ongoing needs for assistance from and to National Health Service (NHS) partners or other agencies
- equipment and re-stocking of supplies.

12.3 Support mechanisms for staff

Staff should be offered a range of support following a major incident. Some of the support mechanisms that could be offered include:

- support from fellow staff members
- support from managers
- access to support via helplines
- access to counselling
- encouragement of a 'no blame' culture
- psychological intervention, including large group therapy, defusing and individual crisis intervention
- access to Occupational Health for the follow-up and aftercare of staff and their families.

12.4 Organisational debriefing

12.4.1 Ground rules when debriefing

It is vital that debriefing is carried out in a way that is conducive to promoting organisational learning and encouraging a 'no blame' culture. Arney (2000) suggests the following ground rules when debriefing:

- conduct the debriefing openly and honestly
- pursue personal, group or organisational understanding and learning

- be consistent with professional responsibilities
- respect the rights of individuals
- value equally all those concerned.

12.4.2 The 'hot' debrief

The key aspects of a 'hot' debrief are as follows:

- it is held immediately after the incident response is completed
- it should address key health and safety issues
- it provides an opportunity to thank staff and provide positive feedback
- it may be facilitated by a range of people from within the Trust
- a number of hot debriefs may be held within a Trust simultaneously following an incident. Each department/unit may wish to hold its own hot debrief to address key issues within their locality.

12.4.3 The Trust debrief

The key aspects of a Trust debrief are as follows:

- it should be held within four weeks of the incident
- it should involve key players within the Trust who were involved in the response to the incident
- it should address organisational issues, not personal or psychological issues
- it should look for both strengths and weaknesses and ideas for future learning
- it provides an opportunity to thank staff and provide positive feedback
- it may be facilitated by a range of people within the Trust.

12.4.4 The multi-agency debrief

If a multi-agency debrief is convened, the key aspects are as follows:

- it should be held within six weeks of the incident
- it should address organisational issues, not personal or psychological issues
- it should look for both strengths and weaknesses and ideas for future learning
- it provides an opportunity to thank staff and provide positive feedback
- it may be facilitated by either the Regional Health Emergency Planning Adviser (RHEPA) or by a partner agency, e.g. the Police Service or a local authority.

12.5 Actions and activities following debriefing

Once debriefing has been completed, there are a number of activities that need to be undertaken (refer to Figure 12.1), including:

- the Trust report
- lessons identified from the incident
- an action plan for the Trust.

As part of this process, it is vital that the Trust identifies a named person to take responsibility for collating and storing all the records, reports and logs.

12.5.1 The Trust report

The Trust report should be completed after the hot debrief and Trust debrief have been finalised. It should:

- summarise the sequence of events
- identify the individuals involved
- describe the actions of your staff
- provide an accurate timeline.

In addition, the report should be:

- factual
- concise
- objective
- blame free.

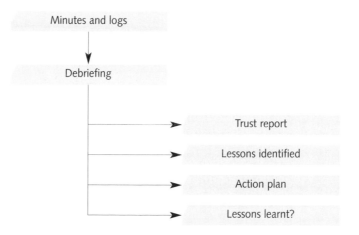

Figure 12.1 Activities following debriefing

12.5.2 Lessons identified

Following the production of a Trust report, the Trust should be able to:

- demonstrate where the response:
  - was effective
  - was not effective
- establish why this was the case at corporate level – objectively
- recommend ways in which to use this information to improve future response
- resist a critique of individual actions
- encourage a 'no blame' culture.

12.5.3 The action plan

Once the lessons have been identified for the Trust, an action plan should be drawn up, against a time frame, to ensure any actions are completed in a timely fashion.

The major incident plan should be reviewed and any amendments, changes or additions to the plan should be included in the action plan, with a time frame to ensure the changes are introduced in a timely fashion.

The Trust should ensure that a named individual is responsible for the completion of each action within an agreed time frame. Review dates should be set and progress should be documented.

12.5.4 Documents generated

The documents generated from the incident and the recovery phases are:

- incident logs
- minutes of:
  - hot debrief (notes)
  - Trust debrief
  - multi-agency debrief (if convened)
- the Trust report
- lessons identified
- action plan.

12.6 Final steps of the debriefing process

12.6.1 Dissemination

Once the Trust report has been completed, a copy should be sent to:

- Trust Chief Executive
- Strategic Health Authority (SHA): Performance Management
- RHEPA.

12.6.2 Exercising

Once the actions in the action plan are completed, the Trust should start planning the following exercises (in an appropriate time frame) to test the plan:

- a communications exercise
- a tabletop exercise
- a live exercise.

12.6.3 Lessons learnt?

Have the lessons been learnt?

Sadly, learning lessons from a major incident is not as simple as putting ticks in the correct boxes – the lessons must have been identified, the action plan completed, and the plan tested by exercising. Then, only when past mistakes are not repeated, can the lessons be considered to have been learnt.

Has your Trust learnt the lessons from past experience of major incidents?

12.7 Summary

This chapter has provided an overview of debriefing and reporting considerations for a Trust during recovery, as well as some of the support mechanisms that should be made available to staff following a major incident. The hot debrief, the Trust debrief and the multi-agency debrief are identified in the chapter as three types of organisational debriefing which can be used to promote post-event learning. The process of report writing, and the reviewing of plans following the debriefing process, has also been explored.

Annexes

Annex 1: Acute Trust Self-Assessment Checklist

This checklist has been developed as a guide to assist those responsible for the development and monitoring of hospital major incident plans. The checklist draws upon requirements set out in the *Planning for Major Incidents: The NHS Guidance* and the Emergency Planning Standard 25, and for response to mass casualty incidents, including chemical, biological, radiological or nuclear (CBRN) incidents.

Name of Trust: _____ Plan version date:_____ Plan review date:_____

Chief Executive: _____

Executive lead:_____EPLO:_____

Date of assessment: _____

Overall regional comments and feedback:

_____

_____

Assessment criteria used

Does the plan:

	Questions	Yes	No	Partially	Comments
1	Reference all other emergency plans or policies that support the hospital major incident plan?				
2	Provide for endorsement by the Trust?				
3	Set out the responsibilities of the Chief Executive?				
4	Identify somebody responsible for ensuring that the plan is updated, distributed and tested on a regular basis?				
5	Set out the mechanism for consultation across the Trust and with external agencies to validate the plan?				
6	Have version controls within it to ensure that the user has the latest version?				
7	State clearly the circumstances that would constitute a major incident for the hospital?				
8	Set out the alerting arrangements for both external and self declared incidents?				
9	Set out responsibilities for implementing the plan?				
10	Include 24-hour arrangements for alerting managers and other key staff?				
11	Set out the responsibilities of key staff in the hospital?				
12	Identify as key staff people appropriately trained to meet these responsibilities?				
13	Incorporate clear action cards/lists to support key staff in meeting their responsibilities?				
14	Contain arrangements for promptly alerting and establishing a Control Team?				
15	Identify the location and facilities of the Hospital Control Centre?				
16	Set out the mechanism for informing upwards that the Plan has been activated?				
17	Provide an assessment of local hazards and risks?				
18	Set out appropriate Health and Safety measures that staff should be aware of?				
19	Cover the provision of personal protective equipment (PPE) for staff?				
20	Consider the need for a single entry point for all casualties of the incident?				
21	Identify the receiving wards that may need to be used?				

	Questions	Yes	No	Partially	Comments
22	Contain details of communication systems, including any radios for use in major incidents?				
23	Set out arrangements for accommodating the Ambulance Liaison Officer?				
24	Set out arrangements for accommodating the Police Documentation Team (including dedicated fax facilities)?				
25	Detail arrangements for deployment of a Medical Incident Officer to the scene of an incident?				
26	Detail arrangements for deployment of a Mobile Medical Team to the scene of an incident?				
27	Detail arrangements for discharge of patients to increase capacity?				
28	Detail arrangements for transfer of patients or services to other hospitals?				
29	Set out arrangements for meeting the needs of friends and relatives?				
30	Cover provision of counselling and follow-up arrangements for patients and relatives?				
31	Provide for the involvement of VAS/ministers/community leaders/chaplains?				
32	Set out arrangements for dealing with enquiries from the public and the media?				
33	Include arrangements for keeping staff informed of the incident response?				
34	Cover arrangements for staff welfare, including debriefing and counselling?				
35	Make provision for additional mortuary facilities for casualties who die en route to the hospital or soon after arrival?				
36	Make provision for the preservation of forensic evidence?				
37	Identify means to access specialist advice and assistance?				
38	Identify means to access key supplies?				
39	Contain arrangements for dealing with VIP visits following a major incident?				
40	Cover arrangements for recording messages received, management decisions and actions taken during a major incident?				
41	Outline arrangements to support and maintain routine services during a major incident?				
42	Set out arrangements with other hospitals/agencies for receiving/providing support?				
43	Cover the special arrangements needed in the event that children are involved in an incident?				
44	Address how the hospital will manage a mass casualty incident where routine emergency resources and facilities are inadequate?				
45	Cover specific arrangements for dealing with a chemical, biological, radiological or nuclear incident?				
46	Cover arrangements and facilities for decontamination of casualties from a chemical, biological, radiological or nuclear incident where potential contamination is identified before entry to the hospital?				
47	Set out arrangements for preventing contamination of the A&E Department by self-referring patients following a chemical, biological, or radiological incident?				
48	Set out arrangements for mitigating the effects if part of the hospital becomes contaminated?				
49	Set out the arrangements for accessing stocks of antidotes/vaccines?				

Additional comments/good practice:

(Department of Health 2002a)

Annex 2: Primary Care Trust Self-Assessment Checklist

Name of Trust: _____Plan version date:_____ Plan review date:_____

Chief Executive: _____

Executive lead:_____EPLO:_____

Date of assessment: _____

Overall regional comments and feedback: _____

_____

Assessment criteria used

	Questions	Yes	No	Partially	Comments
1	Is there Executive Board level ownership of the plan and supporting processes? Has the plan been signed off by the Chief Executive of the PCT?				
2	Is it clear from the plan that mechanisms are in place for ensuring that appropriate planning takes place, e.g. planning group, multi-agency group, etc?				
3	Is there a clear statement as to what constitutes a major incident?				
4	Does the plan include statements about mass casualty situations? Is it clear from the plan how 'scale up' can occur?				
5	Does the plan include mechanisms for accessing the National Reserve National Stock – pods?				
6	Does the plan take account of all latest Department of Health guidance?				
7	Are there clear alerting procedures? Is it clear who has responsibility for alerting and calling in appropriate personnel?				
8	Are the Local Health Protection arrangements detailed in the plan and is it clear who is the lead PCT and which PCTs they are leading on behalf of?				
9	Is it clear within the plan that all stakeholders and external agencies have been involved in drawing up the arrangements?				
10	Has the local Ambulance Trust been involved in agreeing the plans?				
11	Are roles and responsibilities within the plan clear and explicit?				
12	Have staff been trained to ensure that they know what their role and responsibilities are?				
13	Does the plan incorporate action cards – if so are they clear and do they support the roles identified within the plan?				
14	Are the duties of the Chief Executives clearly defined and their responsibilities in the event of a major incident clear?				
15	Is it clear who will be responsible for coordination and management of widespread incidents contained within the Strategic Health Authority (SHA) geographical boundary?				
16	Is it clear within the plan who will attend Police Gold control in the event that wider strategic management of an incident becomes necessary?				
17	Does the plan identify clear procedures for dealing with an internal major incident – business continuity plans for loss of own infrastructure?				
18	Is it clear from the plan what constitutes an internal major incident?				
19	Is the location of the control centre clearly stated and are the arrangements detailed in the plan?				
20	Can this facility be set up in and out of hours?				

Questions	Yes	No	Partially	Comments
Communication arrangements				
21 Is it clear within the plan how communication arrangements will work at PCT level and across the health protection network?				
22 Does the plan include out of hour arrangements?				
23 Is it clear how urgent messages and health alerts will be transmitted across the health economy in and out of hours?				
24 Are there robust arrangements for dealing with the media?				
25 Is it clear who will lead the media response for the PCT and how the response fits into the wider multi-agency mechanisms?				
26 Does the media response incorporate how to inform the public in the event that health advice might need to be given to a whole locality?				
27 Is there provision in the plan for a 24-hour media response?				
28 Is it clear how the SHA will be informed of incidents? This should include arrangements for briefing the SHA.				
29 Is it clear within the plan how regional arrangements can be accessed?				
30 Does the plan incorporate arrangements in the event of chemical, biological, radiological or nuclear (CBRN) incidents?				
31 Are the arrangements to convene a Joint Health Advisory Cell (JHAC) specifically detailed?				
32 Is it clear who within the PCT/Local Health Protection arrangements is responsible for the formation of a JHAC? For example, Director of Public Health, or Consultant in Communicable Disease Control (CCDC) or Regional Health Emergency Planning Adviser (Regional HEPA).				
33 Does the plan cover chemical incidents?				
34 Is it clear within the plan who needs to be contacted in the event of a chemical incident and is CHMRC's number in the plan?				
35 Does the plan cover infectious disease outbreaks?				
36 Does the plan include radiation incident arrangements?				
37 Is it clear within the plan who the PCT can ask for advice in and out of hours for a range of incidents?				
38 Is there mention of debriefing and follow-up arrangements, including counselling and support to patients, relatives and staff?				
39 Is there a nominated Emergency Planning Officer who is responsible for ensuring the plan is updated, tested and disseminated?				
40 Does the plan have an end of shelf life date that acts as a reminder to update the plan?				
41 Is there obvious version control within the document to ensure assurance that the user has the latest version?				
42 Is there a mechanism for promptly informing the SHA and Regional Health Protection Agency teams that plans have been activated?				

Additional comments/good practice:

(Department of Health 2002a)

Annex 3: Ambulance Trust Self-Assessment Checklist

Name of Trust: _____Plan version date:_____Plan review date:_____

Chief Executive: _____

Executive lead:_____EPLO:_____

Date of assessment: _____

Overall comments and feedback: _____

_____

Assessment criteria (CA ref relates to the Emergency Preparedness Controls Assurance Standard)

The plan is up to date

CA ref	Questions:	Yes	No	Partially	Document ref	Comments
10/11	**(a) Plan is part of a continuous process**					
5/6/7 /12	Evidence of ownership by a specific post-holder for the process of formulation, testing, review and amendment of the Trust's emergency/major incident plans					
6/7 /11 /12	Evidence that mechanisms are in place for ensuring that appropriate planning takes place within an appropriate structure – e.g. planning group, regular reporting at board level (including independent audit)					
6/11	Evidence of amendment records, a statement as to when the plan was last updated and by whom					
6	Evidence that the plan is regularly reviewed, updated and tested					
6	Evidence of version control and of a style conducive to a continuous process					
6	Evidence of a statement to say plan is under constant review					
4	Evidence that clearly details the distribution of the plan (extracts) including circulation to NHS and external agencies					
1	Evidence of endorsement by Chief Executive					
1/2	**(b) Plan incorporates up-to-date national guidance**					
8	Evidence of references to relevant guidance/legislation					
1/2/3	Evidence of references to other relevant plans and/or policies that support the Trust response to an incident					
8	Evidence of references to national guidance/briefing (particularly: mass casualty; chemical incidents response; public health response to deliberate release of biological and chemical agents)					

The plan incorporates all elements of the Trust's response as outlined in national guidance

1/2	A clear statement of the Trust role and responsibilities in the event of a major incident/emergency					
1/2	Clear arrangements identifying responsibilities and authority for implementing the plan					
1/2	Clear alerting and activating procedures for both internal and external incidents					
1/2	Evidence that the emergency response arrangements are integrated into the organisation's everyday working structure and processes					
1	Clear statements of the roles and responsibilities of key staff/functions, including Chief Executive					
1/2	Clear arrangements for the alerting and recall of key staff (24-hour coverage) and identifies those to be contacted					
2/3/4	Clearly sets out communications pathways, both internal and external (including arrangements for keeping staff informed)					
1/2	Clear arrangements for establishing an incident management team					
1/2	Clear arrangements for the maintenance of documentation and logs					
1/2	Clear arrangements for establishment of functional management at incident location					
1/23 /4	Clear arrangements for coordinating NHS communications at the scene					
3	Arrangements for creating additional capacity including staff recall and mutual aid arrangements (such arrangements must also reflect the possibility of acting in support of other Ambulance Trusts)					
7	Clear arrangements for obtaining and transporting Mobile Medical Teams					
2	Clear arrangements for special needs of children					

CA ref	Questions:	Yes	No	Partially	Document ref	Comments
2	Clear procedures for initial triage					
3/4/5 /6/7/8	Arrangements for the health and safety of all NHS personnel deployed to the incident site					
2	Clear evidence of command and control arrangements within the health economy and unambiguous reporting lines (linkage to lead Primary Care Trust (PCT), Strategic Health Authority (SHA) and Department of Health (DH)					
1/2	Action cards/lists for key staff/functions					
11/12	Evidence that action cards are regularly reviewed and updated					
2/3	Clear instructions regarding the preservation of forensic evidence					
2/3	Arrangements for monitoring system pressure points					
1/2/3	Outline arrangements for business continuity					
2	Clear arrangements for visiting VIPs					
2	Sets out clear arrangements for dealing with enquiries from the media (including corporate NHS and multi-agency involvement)					
7	Clear identification of access arrangements for resources required for the response including: additional staff, communications systems, vehicles, plant, etc.					
7	Sets out arrangements for support facilities, supplies, voluntary aid societies, etc.					
2	Arrangements for the welfare, debriefing and where required subsequent psychological support for staff					
7	Clear arrangements in the event of communications failure and transport disruption					
1/2/3	Clear provision for the support of the strategic coordination of the NHS within the health economy (this should include arrangements for attendance at multi-agency coordinating group and if required participation in the JHAC)					
2/3	Clear mechanism for activation of the plan in response to widespread incidents, for which the SHA has responsibility for NHS coordination					

The plan is flexible enough to meet all possible causes of a major incident

CA ref	Questions:	Yes	No	Partially	Document ref	Comments
2/3/6	Clearly define and cover both external and internal incidents and identified risks/hazards. Where the plan does not cover internal incidents there are references to separate contingency plans					
2	Evidence that internal/external risks and hazards are regularly reviewed					
3	Plan specific arrangements for chemical, biological, radioactive and nuclear incidents, including the provision of personal protective equipment and decontamination arrangements					
3	In support of Acute Trusts, sets out arrangements and facilities for decontamination of casualties, where potential contamination is identified before entry to the hospital					
2/3	Clearly identifies the arrangements to access specialist advice relating to chemical, biological, radioactive and nuclear incidents					
3	Evidence of specific arrangements to deal with mass casualty incidents, relative to capacity management plans and mutual aid arrangements					
3	Identifies the arrangements for access to specialist supplies, e.g. National Reserve Stocks (pods)					

The plan is clear, unambiguous and easy to use

CA ref	Questions:	Yes	No	Partially	Document ref	Comments
1/2	Easy-to-read language and format					
1/2/3	Plan has comprehensive index, cross-referenced as appropriate					
1	Action cards/lists are simple, prioritised and accessible					
1	Does not require users unnecessarily to access other documents and references or refer them to annexes					
1/2	Plan is brief and concise containing key information only					

Plan states relationship to external organisations (including NHS), their respective roles and how the organisations will interface with each other

CA ref	Questions:	Yes	No	Partially	Document ref	Comments
4	A statement of other key organisations and their roles					
4	An indication of robust liaison arrangements and procedures to facilitate multi-agency coordination					
4	Evidence of liaison and mutual aid arrangements with other elements of the NHS					
4	Evidence that other key organisations, both NHS and external agencies, have been consulted during the formulation of the plan for validation purposes					

Additional comments/examples of good practice:

Annex 4: Societies and Institutes

British Association of Public Safety Communications Officers (BAPCO)

WWW   www.bapco.org.uk

Address   Ken Mott (CEO),
PO Box 374,
Lincoln LN1 1FY

Telephone   01522 575542

Fax   01522 575542

Email   enquiries@bapco.org.uk

Business Continuity Institute (BCI) UK

WWW   www.thebci.org

Address   PO Box 4474,
Worcester WR6 5YA

Telephone   0870 603 8783

Fax   0870 603 8761

Email   thebci@btinternet.com

Emergency Planning Society (EPS) UK

WWW   www.emergplansoc.org.uk

Address   Northumberland House,
11 The Pavement,
Popes Lane,
London W5 4NG

Telephone   020 8579 7971

Fax   020 8579 7972

Email   HQ@emergplansoc.org.uk

Institute of Civil Defence and Disaster Studies (ICDDS) UK

WWW   www.icdds.org

Address   PO Box 698,
Camberley,
Surrey GU15 3WY

Fax   020 7173 6001 (contact: Charles van Oppen)

Institute of Emergency Management

WWW   www.iem.org

Address   PO Box 271,
Hatfield,
Hertfordshire AL10 9ZT

Telephone   01707 284158

Fax   01707 284170

Email   e.dykes@herts.ac.uk

Society of Industrial Emergency Services Officers (SIESO) UK

WWW	www.sieso.org.uk
Address	Secretary SIESO,
	The Oaks,
	Thames Lane,
	Cricklade,
	Wiltshire SN6 6BH
Telephone	01793 759225
Email	sec@sieso.org.uk

World Association for Disaster and Emergency Medicine (WADEM)

WWW	www.wadem.medicine.wisc.edu
Address	WADEM,
	732 N. Midvale Blvd,
	Suite 201,
	Madison WI 53705
	USA
Telephone	+1 608 236 2069
Fax	+1 608 265 3037
Email	mlb@medicine.wisc.edu

Annex 5: Government Departments and Agencies

Department for Environment, Food and Rural Affairs (Defra)

WWW   www.defra.gov.uk

Address   Information Resource Centre,
Lower Ground Floor,
Ergon House,
c/o Nobel House,
17 Smith Square,
London SW1P 3JR

Telephone 020 7238 6951

Email   helpline@defra.gsi.gov.uk

Department of Health

WWW   www.dh.gov.uk

Address   79 Whitehall,
London SW1A 2NS

Telephone 020 7210 4850 (10 a.m. to 4 p.m.)

Switchboard 020 7210 3000

Email   dhmail@dh.gsi.gov.uk

Department of Trade and Industry

WWW   www.dti.gov.uk

Address   1 Victoria Street,
London SW1H 0ET

Telephone 020 7215 5000

Email   Enquiries@dti.gsi.gov.uk

Department for Transport

WWW   www.dft.gov.uk

Address   Great Minister House,
76 Marsham Street,
London SW1P 4DR

Telephone 020 7944 8300

Drinking Water Inspectorate

WWW   www.dwi.gov.uk

Address   Ashdown House,
123 Victoria Street,
London SW1E 6DE

Telephone 020 7944 5956

Environment Agency

WWW	www.environment-agency.gov.uk
Address	Rio House,
	Aztec West,
	Almondsbury,
	Bristol BS32 4UD
Telephone	0845 933 3111
Email	enquiries@environment-agency.gov.uk

Food Standards Agency

WWW	www.foodstandards.gov.uk
Email	helpline@foodstandards.gsi.gov.uk

Food Standards Agency – England

Address	Aviation House,
	125 Kingsway,
	London WC2B 6NH
Telephone	020 7276 8000

Food Standards Agency – Scotland

Address	Floor 6,
	St Magnus House,
	25 Guild Street,
	Aberdeen AB11 8NJ
Telephone	01224 285100

Food Standards Agency – Wales

Address	Floor 1,
	Southgate House,
	Wood Street,
	Cardiff CF10 1EW
Telephone	02920 678999

Health and Safety Executive

WWW	www.hse.gov.uk
Address	Rose Court,
	2 Southwark Bridge,
	London SE1 9HS
Help line	08701 545500
Switchboard	020 7717 6000
Email	hseinformationservices@natbrit.com

Health Protection Agency

WWW   www.hpa.org.uk

Address   Health Protection Agency Central Office,
Floor 7,
Holburn Gate,
330 High Holburn,
London WC1V 7PP

Telephone   020 7759 2700

Ministry of Defence

WWW   www.mod.uk

Address   The Ministerial Correspondence Unit,
Room 222,
The Old War Office,
Whitehall,
London SW1A 2HB

Telephone   0870 607 4455

National Chemical Emergency Centre

WWW   www.the-ncec.com

Address   Culham,
Abingdon,
Oxfordshire OX14 3ED

Telephone   01235 463060

Email   ncec@aeat.co.uk

Scottish Centre for Infection and Environmental Health

WWW   www.show.scot.nhs.uk/scieh/

Address   Clifton House,
Clifton Place,
Glasgow G3 7LN

Telephone   0141 300 1100

Fax   0141 300 1170

Scottish Executive

WWW   www.scotland.gov.uk

Address   The Scottish Executive Health Department,
St Andrew's House,
Regent Road,
Edinburgh EH1 3DG

General
inquiry line   0845 774 1741

Fax   0131 244 8240

Email   ceu@scotland.gov.uk

National Assembly for Wales

WWW	www.wales.gov.uk/index.htm
Address	Cardiff Bay,
	Cardiff CF99 1NA
Telephone	02920 825111

Other agencies

British Association for Counselling and Psychotherapy (BACP)

WWW	www.bacp.co.uk
Address	BACP House,
	35–37 Albert Street,
	Rugby CV21 2SG
Telephone	01788 550899
Email	bacp@bacp.co.uk

Fire Service Training College

WWW	www.fireservicecollege.ac.uk
Address	Fire Research Establishment,
	London Road,
	Moreton-in-the-Marsh,
	Gloucester GL56 0RH
Telephone	01608 650831
Email	enquiries@fireservicecollege.ac.uk

Meteorological Office

WWW	www.met-office.gov.uk
Address	London Road,
	Bracknell,
	Berkshire RG12 2SZ
Telephone	01344 420242
Email	enquiries@metoffice.com

Voluntary agencies

British Association for Immediate Care (BASICS)

WWW	www.basics.org.uk
Address	Turret House,
	Turret Lane,
	Ipswich IP4 1DL
Telephone	0870 165 4999
Fax	0870 165 4949
Email	admin@basics.org.uk

British Red Cross

WWW	www.redcross.org.uk
Address	National House,
	9 Grosvenor Crescent,
	London SW1X 7EJ
Telephone	020 7235 5454
Email	information@redcross.org.uk

St. John Ambulance Brigade Headquarters

WWW	www.sja.org.uk
Address	Edwina Mountbatten House,
	63 York Street,
	London W1H 1PS
Telephone	020 7258 3456
Email	Districthq@london.sja.org.uk

Woman's Royal Voluntary Service (WRVS)

WWW	www.wrvs.org.uk
Address	Milton Hill House,
	Milton Hill,
	Abingdon,
	Oxfordshire OX13 6AD
Telephone	01235 442900
Email	Enquiries@wrvs.org.uk

Annex 6: Websites

National sources

Department of Health   www.dh.gov.uk

This is the website of the unit within the Department of Health responsible for emergency planning. The site contains specific information for action in the event of a major incident.

Environment Agency   www.environment-agency.gov.uk

This is the public agency responsible for the protection of the environment for England and Wales.

Health Protection Agency   www.hpa.org.uk

The website of the national agency responsible for health and safety of England and Wales. A list of the various organisations within the HPA is available, as well as links to information on infectious diseases, chemicals and poisons, radiation, local services and emergency response.

Health and Safety Executive   www.hse.gov.uk

This is the agency responsible for health and safety issues arising in the work environment. The website contains extensive links to other agencies, both national and international, involved in workplace safety. There are links to reports and regulations that govern workplace health and safety.

Home Office   www.homeoffice.gov.uk

The website of the governmental agency responsible for management of internal affairs for England and Wales. Links to most government regulation texts and other governmental agencies are available.

London Emergency Services Liaison Panel   www.leslp.gov.uk

In-depth information on steps to take in a major incident, including the role of the emergency services, defining and declaring a major incident, interaction between different agencies and media liaison issues. The site contains the downloadable LESLP manual in PDF format and links to some other governmental agencies.

London Prepared   www.londonprepared.gov.uk

This website details emergency preparation and planning for London and has direct links to the UK Resilience website. Numerous London links to governmental and non-governmental agencies are available, including police services, the Environment Agency, transport and travel authorities, and news and information links.

Medical Toxicology Unit   www.medtox.org

The website of the Medical Toxicology Unit of Guy's and St Thomas' Hospital. Contains information about toxicology, poisons and chemical incidents.

UK Resilience   www.ukresilience.info/home.htm

Provides information and links to a variety of governmental and non-governmental agencies that are involved in emergency situations in the UK. Civil contingencies, providing information on a variety of crises, are grouped according to type of incident (e.g. aviation, food alerts, chemical accidents, etc.).

International sources

Awareness and Preparedness for Emergencies at Local Level
www.unepie.org/pc/apell/home.html

Website of the programme designed by United Nations Environment Program (UNEP) to facilitate interaction between various agencies in the prevention of accidents. The website contains links to the major international and regional agencies involved in disaster management and prevention.

Emergency Management Australia   www.ema.gov.au

This website contains sections on preparing for unexpected events, and information on disasters for the community and lessons learnt in previous incidents. Links to the Australian Journal of Emergency Management and the Australian federal government agencies involved in disaster management are available.

US Environmental Protection Agency   www.epa.gov

The website contains information pertaining to the protection of human health and the safeguarding of the natural environment. A large amount of information on various environmental issues, including emergency planning, is detailed under the EPA topics.

Federal Emergency Management Agency   www.fema.gov

The website of the US Department of Homeland Security, providing up-to-date news features and a library section of practical information for use during emergency situations, as well as links to other state offices and agencies in the USA.

Ministry of Civil Defence and Emergency Management, New Zealand
www.civildefence.govt.nz

This website contains sections giving information for the public as well as comprehensive information on emergency management and the requirements of the Civil Defence and Emergency Management Act 2002. Resource documents and links are also available.

Natural Hazards Center at University of Colorado, Boulder, USA
www.colorado.edu/hazards

The Natural Hazards Center is a national and international centre for information on natural hazards and human adjustments to hazards and disasters. The website provides an extensive source of information regarding disasters, including the 'quick response reports' series, detailing research done immediately after major incidents.

World Health Organisation   www.who.int/en

The website offers specific information for individual countries, as well as an extensive A to Z list of a variety of health topics, including emergency policies. The focus is on biological/disease-related health issues.

Annex 7: Universities and Colleges offering courses in Emergency Management

Coventry University

WWW   www.cov.ac.uk

Address   Centre for Disaster Management,

               Coventry University,

               Priory Street,

               Coventry CV1 5FB

Telephone   024 7688 7688

Fax   024 7688 8257

Emergency Planning College

WWW   www.epcollege.gov.uk

Address   Emergency Planning College,

               The Hawkhills,

               Easingwold,

               York YO61 3EG

Telephone   01347 821406

Fax   01347 822575

Lincoln University

WWW   www.lincoln.ac.uk

Address   Faculty of Health, Life and Social Sciences,

               Brayford Pool,

               Lincoln LN6 7TS

Telephone   01522 886852

Fax   01522 886791

Northumbria University

WWW   www.northumbria.ac.uk

Address   Division of Geography and Environmental Management,

               Lipman Building,

               Sandyford Road,

               Newcastle-upon-Tyne NE1 8ST

Telephone   0191 227 3951

Fax   0191 227 4715

University of Birmingham

WWW   www.bham.ac.uk/ipeh

Address   Division of Environmental Health and Risk Management,

               Public Health Building,

               University of Birmingham,

               Edgbaston,

               Birmingham B15 2TT

Telephone   0121 414 6756

Fax   0121 414 3077

University of Central Lancashire

WWW	www.uclan.ac.uk
Address	Department of Environmental Management,
	University of Central Lancashire,
	Preston PR1 2HE
Telephone	01772 893496
Fax	01772 892926

University of Hertfordshire

WWW	www.herts.ac.uk
Address	Civil Emergency Management Centre,
	College Lane,
	Hatfield,
	Hertfordshire AL10 9AB
Telephone	07956 135580
Fax	01707 284170

University of Leeds

WWW	www.leeds.ac.uk
Address	University of Leeds,
	Leeds LS2 9JT
Telephone	0113 243 1751
Fax	0113 244 3923

University of Leicester

WWW	www.le.ac.uk/scarman
Address	The Scarman Centre,
	University of Leicester,
	The Friars,
	154 Upper New Walk,
	Leicester LE1 7QA
Telephone	0116 252 5730
Fax	0116 252 5788
Email	aem5@le.ac.uk

University of Manchester

WWW	www.man.ac.uk
Address	University of Manchester,
	School of Epidemiology and Health Sciences,
	The Medical School,
	Oxford Road,
	Manchester M13 9PT
Telephone	0161 275 5201
Fax	0161 275 7712

University of Portsmouth

WWW	www.port.ac.uk/departments/sees
Address	University of Portsmouth,
	Faculty of Environment,
	School of Environmental Design and Management,
	Portland Building,
	Portland Street,
	Portsmouth PO1 3AH
Telephone	02392 842931
Fax	02392 842913

University of Southampton

WWW	www.soton.ac.uk
Address	University of Southampton,
	Highfield,
	Southampton SO17 1BJ
Telephone	023 8059 3076
Fax	023 8059 3285
Email	mmtmail8@soton.ac.uk

University of Teeside

WWW	www.tees.ac.uk
Address	School of Science and Technology,
	University of Teeside,
	Middlesbrough TS1 3BA
Telephone	01642 342449
Fax	01642 342401

Annex 8: CHALETS and METHANE Mnemonics

CHALETS

C	Casualties, number and severity
H	Hazards, present and potential
A	Access to scene and egress route
L	Location, exact (grid reference)
E	Emergency services, present and required
T	Type of incident
S	Safety

(Waspe 2003)

METHANE

M	Major incident	*Standby or declared*
E	Exact location	*Grid reference*
T	Type of incident	*Rail, chemical, road*
H	Hazards	*Present or potential*
A	Access	*Direction of approach*
N	Number of casualties	*And their severity/type*
E	Emergency services	*Present or required*

(Rowe 2003)

Glossary

Where appropriate, the following definitions are extracted from either the Department of Health document (1998), *Planning for Major Incidents*, the Home Office document (2003), *Dealing with Disaster* or the London Emergency Services Liaison Panel (LESLP)(2003) publication, *Major Incident Procedure Manual*. The glossary provides some of the key terms used not only in this publication but also in emergency planning and response environments.

KEY

▲   Denotes a definition provided by the Department of Health (1998).
✳   Denotes a definition taken from LESLP (2003).
All other definitions are taken from Home Office (2003), unless otherwise stated.

A

ACCOLC	Access Overload Control (for cellular radio telephones). The Access Overload Control scheme gives call preference to registered essential users on the four main mobile networks in the UK, if the scheme is invoked during a major emergency.
Ambulance Incident Officer (AIO)	The officer of the Ambulance Service with overall responsibility for the work of that service at the scene of a major incident. Works in close liaison with the Medical Incident Officer (MIO) to ensure effective use of the medical and ambulance resources at the scene.
Ambulance loading point	An area, preferably hard standing, in close proximity to the casualty clearing station, where ambulances can be manoeuvred and patients placed on board for transfer to hospital. Helicopter landing provision may also be needed.
Ambulance Safety Officer (ASO)	The officer responsible for monitoring operations and ensuring the safety of personnel working under his/her control within the inner cordon at the major incident site. Liaises with safety officers from other emergency services. ▲
Ante mortem data	Information obtained from family, friends, etc. about a person who is believed to be among the deceased.
Ante mortem team	Officers responsible for liaising with the next of kin on all matters relating to the identification of the deceased.

B

Bellwin scheme	Discretionary scheme for providing central government financial assistance in exceptional circumstances to affected local authorities in the event of a major emergency.
Body holding area/Body collection point	An area close to the scene where the dead can be temporarily held until transfer to the temporary mortuary or mortuary.
Bronze level	Operational commander.

C

Cascade system	System whereby one person or organisation calls out others who in turn initiate further call-outs as necessary.

Casualty	A person killed or physically or mentally injured in war, accident or civil emergency. For Casualty Bureau purposes the term encompasses any person involved in an incident, including evacuees. In maritime emergencies, it is also used to refer to a vessel in distress.
Casualty Bureau	Police central contact and information point for all records and data relating to casualties, evacuees and others affected by the incident.
Casualty Clearing Officer	The ambulance officer who, in liaison with the Medical Incident Officer, ensures an efficient patient throughput at the casualty clearing station.
Casualty clearing station	An area set up at a major incident by the Ambulance Service, in liaison with the Medical Incident Officer, to assess, triage and treat casualties and direct their evacuation.
Casualty label	Colour-coded label used by Ambulance Service and medical teams to identify the priority of a casualty. ▲
CHEMET	A scheme administered by the Meteorological Office, providing information on weather conditions as they affect an incident involving hazardous chemicals.
CIMAH/ COMAH sites	Industrial sites which are subject to the Control of Industrial Major Accident Hazards Regulations 1984. From February 1999, these were replaced by the Control of Major Accident Hazards Regulations. ▲
Civil Contingencies Committee (CCC)	Committee of ministers (chaired normally by the Home Secretary) convened to provide central government oversight of a major emergency.
Civil Contingencies coordination	The Cabinet Office secretariat which provides the central focus for the cross-departmental and cross-agency commitment, and cooperation that will enable the UK to deal effectively with disruptive challenges and crises.
Command	The authority for an agency to direct the actions of its own resources (both personnel and equipment).
Control	The authority to direct strategic and tactical operations in order to complete an assigned function. This includes the ability to direct the activities of other agencies engaged in the completion of that function. The control of the assigned function also carries with it a responsibility for the health and safety of those involved.
Control room	Centre for the control of the movements and activities of each emergency service's personnel and equipment. Liaises with the other services' control rooms.
Coordination	The harmonious integration of the expertise of all the agencies involved, with the object of effectively and efficiently bringing the incident to a successful conclusion.
Cordon – inner	Surrounds and protects the immediate scene of an incident.
Cordon – outer	Seals off a controlled area around an incident to which unauthorised persons are not allowed access.

D

Devolved administrations	The Scottish Executive, Welsh Assembly Government and Northern Ireland Executive.

E

Emergency centre/ Emergency control centre	Local authority operations centre from which the management and coordination of local authority incident support is carried out.
Environmental Health Officer (EHO)	A professional officer responsible for assisting people to attain environmental conditions which are conducive to good health. Most EHOs work for local authorities and are concerned with administration, inspection, education and law enforcement. ▲
Evacuation assembly point	Building or area to which evacuees are directed for transfer/transportation to a survivor reception centre or evacuation (or rest) centre.
Evacuation (or rest) centre	Building designated by local authority for temporary accommodation of people evacuated from their homes. See also 'Survivor reception centre'. ▲

F

Forward control point	Each service's command and control facility nearest to the scene of the incident, responsible for immediate direction, deployment and security.
Friends and relatives reception centre	Secure area set aside for the use and the interviewing of friends and relatives arriving at the scene (or other location associated with an incident, such as at an airport or port). Established by the police in consultation with the local authority.

G

Gold level	Strategic commander.

H

Hazard	A hazard is anything that is 'a source of potential harm or a situation with the potential to cause loss' (Emergency Management Australia 2000: 3).
Hazard identification	This is the term used for gathering information about hazards – potential sources of harm/loss within a definable area. The process of identifying hazards is not an exact science, and may be done using an arithmetic process or through simple discussion and research.
Health Advisory Group on Chemical Contamination Incidents (HAGCCI)	A group of experts able to give independent and authoritative advice to the DH on the human health effects of chemical contamination. ▲
Health Protection Agency	The Health Protection Agency is a new, independent organisation dedicated to protecting people's health. It brings together the expertise formerly found in a number of official organisations. ▲
Hospital control team	Team managing a hospital's response to a major incident. ▲

149

Hospital coordination centre	The centre set up at a receiving hospital to manage the in-hospital response: to collate, for internal use, data concerning casualties received (their condition, bed states, theatres available); and to provide information to the police documentation team, as appropriate. ▲
Hospital documentation team	Team of police officers responsible for completing police casualty record cards in hospitals.
Hospital friends and relatives reception centre	An assembly point at a receiving hospital where friends and relatives can be received and arrangements made for their special needs. The receiving hospital is responsible for establishing the centre.

I

Incident control point/Incident control post	The point from which each of the emergency services' tactical managers can control their services' response to a land-based incident. Together, the incident control points form the focal point for coordinating all activities on site. Also referred to as 'Silver control'. In London, incident control points are grouped together to form the Joint Emergency Services Control Centre (JESCC).
Incident Officer	An officer at the scene who commands the tactical response of his/her respective service.
Incident response team	Multi-agency/-disciplinary team which directs action and takes corporate decisions on behalf of the health authority. ▲
Inner cordon	Surrounds and protects the immediate scene of an incident.
Integrated emergency management (IEM)	An approach to preventing and managing emergencies that entails five key activities: assessment, prevention, preparation, response and recovery. IEM is geared to the idea of building greater overall resilience in the face of a broad range of disruptive challenges.
Investigating agencies	Those organisations that are legally empowered to investigate the cause of an accident (Air Accident Investigation Branch, Marine Accident Investigation Branch, HSE, etc.).

J

Joint Emergency Services Control Centre (JESCC)	The main Police Service, Fire Brigade and Ambulance Service control/command units, together with the public utilities and local authority, which should be located close to one another and form the focus point from which the incident will be managed. ✳

L

Lead government department	Department which, in the event of major disaster/emergency, coordinates central government activity.
Local emergency centre (LEC)	Purpose-designed and specially equipped control centre for the coordination of the response to a nuclear emergency emanating from a civil nuclear power station.

M

Major incident
Any emergency that requires the implementation of special arrangements by one or more of the emergency services, the NHS or the local authority. For the NHS, a major incident is any occurrence which presents a serious threat to the health of the community or disruption to the service, or which causes (or is likely to cause) such numbers or types of casualties as to require special arrangements to be implemented by hospitals, Ambulance Services or health authorities. ▲

Major incident control room
Established in protracted emergencies to coordinate the overall response, deal with ongoing resource and logistical requirements, and provide facilities for senior command functions. Often referred to as 'Gold control'.

Major incident procedures
Pre-planned and exercised procedures which are activated once a major incident has been declared.

Marshalling area
Area to which resources and personnel which are not immediately required at the scene, or are being held for further use, can be directed to standby.

Media centre/ Media briefing centre
Central location for media enquiries, providing communication, conference and monitoring facilities, facilities for interviews and briefings, and access to responding organisation personnel. Staffed by spokespersons from all the principal services/organisations responding.

Media Liaison Officer
Representative who has responsibility for liaising with the media on behalf of his/her organisation.

Media liaison point
An area adjacent to the scene, which is designated for the reception and accreditation of media personnel and for briefing on arrangements for reporting, filming and photographing. Staffed by media liaison officers from appropriate services.

Medical Incident Officer (MIO)
Medical officer with overall responsibility (in close liaison with the Ambulance Incident Officer) for the management of medical resources at the scene of a major incident. He/she should not be a member of a Mobile Medical Team.

Mobile Medical Team (MMT)
Nominated hospital personnel, mobilised at the request of the Ambulance Service, who provide on-site treatment.

Mutual aid arrangements
Cross-boundary arrangements under which emergency services, local authorities and other organisations request extra staff and/or equipment for use in a disaster.

N

The National Focus
The National Focus for Work on Response to Chemical Incidents.

NHS Direct
24-hour health telephone helpline, staffed by nurses.

O

Operational (Bronze) level
The operational level of management reflects the normal day-to-day arrangements for responding to smaller scale emergencies. It is the level at which the management of 'hands-on' work is undertaken at the incident site(s) or associated areas.

Outer cordon	Seals off a controlled area around an incident to which unauthorised persons are not allowed access.
Overall Incident Commander (Gold)	The designated senior officer in charge of the police response, who normally coordinates the strategic roles of all the emergency services and other organisations involved.

P

Paramedic	Someone holding a current certificate of proficiency in ambulance paramedical skills issued by or with the approval of the Secretary of State for Health. ▲
Patient group directions (PGDs)	These are documents which make it legal for medicines to be given to groups of patients, e.g. in a mass casualty situation, without individual prescriptions having to be written for each patient. They can also be used to empower staff other than doctors legally to give the medicines in question. ▲
Police Casualty Bureau	Police central contact and information point for all records and data relating to casualties, evacuees and others affected by the incident. ▲
Police documentation team (hospital)	Team of police officers responsible for completing police casualty record cards in hospitals. ▲
Post-mortem data	Information obtained from the post-mortem examination process.
Primary Care Trust (PCT)	With the abolishment of the old health authorities, local Primary Care Trusts (PCTs) have become the lead NHS organisations in assessing need, planning and securing all health services, and improving health in their localities. They also provide most community services and develop primary care services, including GPs and dentists, and they now have responsibility for emergency planning. They are performance managed by the Strategic Health Authorities. ▲

R

Radioactive Incident Monitoring Network (RIMNET)	The national response system (for overseas nuclear accidents) operated by the Department for Transport, Local Government and the Regions. ▲
Receiving hospital(s)	Any hospital selected by the Ambulance Service from those designated by health authorities to receive casualties in the event of a major incident.
Reception arrangements for military patients (RAMP)	Military plan for coping (with NHS help) with military casualties evacuated to the UK from an area of conflict overseas. ▲
Rendezvous point (RVP)	Point to which all resources arriving at the outer cordon are directed for logging, briefing, equipment issue and deployment. In protracted large-scale incidents there may be a need for more than one rendezvous point.
Resilience	Resilience is the ability of an organisation or working practice, etc. to prepare for, respond to and recover from the likely impact of a hazard and associated risks.

Rest centre	Building designated by the local authority for the temporary accommodation of evacuees, with overnight facilities if necessary – see also 'Evacuation (or rest) centre'.
Risk	There are a number of different definitions of risk. For the purpose of this handbook, risk is defined as the likelihood of an identified hazard causing harm (MCDEM 2002).
Risk assessment	The process of identifying and quantifying risks, which can be done in a number of ways. For the purpose of this handbook, the risk assessment process is detailed in terms of frequency and severity.

S

Search and rescue (SAR)	Operations for locating and retrieving persons in distress, providing for their immediate needs and delivering them to a place of safety.
Senior Investigating Officer (SIO)	The senior detective officer appointed by the senior police officer to assume responsibility for all aspects of the police investigation.
Silver level	Tactical commander.
Statutory services	Those services whose responsibilities are laid down in law: for example, police, fire and ambulance services, HM Coastguard and local authorities.
Strategic coordinating group (SCG)	A group, comprising senior officers of appropriate organisations, which aims to achieve effective inter-agency coordination at strategic level. This group should normally be located away from the immediate scene.
Strategic Health Authority (SHA)	The NHS statutory body providing the bridge between the Department of Health and local NHS Trusts and PCTs, to provide strategic leadership and ensure the delivery of improvements in health, well-being and health services locally. ▲
Strategic (Gold) level	A strategic level of management, which establishes a policy and overall management framework within which tactical managers will work. It establishes strategic objectives and aims to ensure long-term resourcing/expertise.
Survivor reception centre	Secure area, set up by the local authority, to which survivors not requiring acute hospital treatment can be taken for short-term shelter, first aid, interview and documentation. See also 'Evacuation (or rest) centre'.

T

Tactical (Silver) level	A tactical level of management, which provides overall management of the response to an emergency. Tactical managers determine priorities in allocating resources, obtain further resources as required, and plan and coordinate when tasks will be undertaken.
Temporary mortuary	Facility accessible from a disaster area, designated for temporary use as a mortuary and adapted for post-mortem examinations.
Territorial departments	The Scotland Office, Northern Ireland Office and Wales Office.

Triage Process of assessment and allocation of priorities by the medical or ambulance staff at the site or casualty clearing station prior to evacuation. Triage may be repeated at intervals and on arrival at a receiving hospital.

U

Utilities Companies providing essential services, e.g. gas, water, electricity, telephones.

V

Voluntary aid societies (VAS) St. John Ambulance, St. Andrew's Ambulance Association and the British Red Cross Society.

Vulnerability Vulnerability defines the 'susceptibility and resilience' (Emergency Management Australia 2000) of a group of individuals, communities, buildings, working practices, etc. to identified hazards.

W

Welfare coordination team A team normally coordinated by the appropriate local authority social services director or deputy, to look after the longer term welfare needs of those affected by disaster. The team may include representatives from other local authority departments, police, faith organisations and appropriate voluntary organisations.

References

Alibek, K. and Handelman, S. (2000), *Biohazard* (Reading: Arrow Books).

Appleby, L. (1999), *Safer Services: National Confidential Inquiry into Suicide and Homicide by People with Mental Illness* (London: The Stationery Office).

Arney, J. (2000), *Structured Debriefing* (Centre for Structured Debriefing course notes).

Bailey, A. (2003), *Personal Communication.*

Cabinet Office (2003), *Dealing with Disaster* (3rd edn) (London: Brodie Publishing Ltd).

Civil Contingencies Act 2004 (Contingency Planning) Regulations 2005 (London: The Stationery Office).

Civil Contingencies Bill 2004 (London: The Stationery Office).

Code of Practice Committee (1997), *Code of Practice* (Glasgow: Code of Practice Committee).

Court, B. (2002), *Letter to Chief Executives of PCTs.*

Deacon, J. and Deacon, B. (1999), *Perception is Reality: Managing the Media when Emergencies Strike* (Bedford: JB Media Management).

Deacon, J. and Deacon, B. (2000), *Media Management: The Essentials* (Bedford: JB Media Management).

Department of Health (1992), *Risk Management in the NHS* (London: Department of Health).

Department of Health (1998), *Planning for Major Incidents: The NHS Guidance* (London: HMSO).

Department of Health (2000), *Deliberate Release of Biological and Chemical Agents: Guidance to Help Plan the Health Service's Response* (London: Department of Health).

Department of Health (2001), *Ambulance Service Standing Operational Procedures: To Support the Deployment of Modesty and Equipment Pods from the UK Reserve National Stock for Major Incidents* (London: Department of Health).

Department of Health (2002a), *An Organisation with a Memory* (London: The Stationery Office).

Department of Health (2002b), *Getting Ahead of the Curve: A Strategy for Combating Infectious Diseases (Including Other Aspects of Health Protection)* (London: Department of Health).

Department of Health (2002c), 'The Primary Care Trust'. In *Planning for Major Incidents: The NHS Guidance* (London: Department of Health), 87–95.

Department of Health (2004), *Handling Major Incidents: An Operational Doctrine* (London: Department of Health/Health Protection Agency).

Department of Health (2005), *The NHS Emergency Planning Guidance* (London: Emergency Preparedness Division, Department of Health).

Doran, A. (2003), *Written Communication to Trusts, PCTs, Strategic Health Authorities in England.*

Eagles, E., Goodfellow, F., Welsh, F. and Murray, V. (2003), *Environmental and Public Health* (London: HMSO).

Emergency Management Australia (2000), *Emergency Risk Management: Applications Guide* (Canberra: Emergency Management Agency).

Fairman, R. et al. (2001), *Chemical Incident Management: Local Authority Environmental Health Officers* (London: The Stationery Office).

Harrison, H., Clarke, S., Wilson, A. and Murray, V. (2002), 'Chemical contamination of health care facilities and staff'. *Chemical Incident Report* 25: 2–5.

Harthman, J. (2002), *Disaster Law, Disaster Finance and the Consequences* (Sheffield: Sheffield City Council).

Health and Safety Executive (2000), *Management of Health and Safety at Work: Management of Health and Safety at Work Regulations 1999 Approved Code of Practice and Guidance* (Sudbury: Health and Safety Executive).

Health and Safety Executive (2002), *Five Steps to Risk Assessment* (INDG163 (Rev1) 01/02).

Heath, R. (1998), *Crisis Management for Managers and Executives: Business Crises – the Definitive Handbook to Reduction, Readiness, Response and Recovery* (London: Financial Times/Pitman Publishing).

Heptonstall, J. and Gent, N. (2005), *CBRN Incidents: Clinical Management and Health Protection* (London: Health Protection Agency).

Home Office (1998), *The Exercise Planner's Guide: A Guide To Testing Emergency Arrangements* (London: HMSO).

Home Office (2000a), *Dealing with Disaster: Comprehensive Guide to Handling Disasters in the UK* (3rd edn) (London: Home Office).

Home Office (2000b), *How Resilient is Your Business to Disaster? A Comprehensive Guide for any Organisation to Survive and Recover from Disaster* (London: Home Office).

Home Office (2003), *Dealing with Disaster* (revised 3rd edn) (London: Brodie Publishing Ltd).

Home Office (2004), *The Decontamination of People Exposed to Chemical, Biological, Radiological or Nuclear (CBRN) Substances or Materials: Strategic National Guidance* (2nd edn) (London: HMSO).

International Atomic Energy Agency (1988), *The Radiological Accident in Gioânia* (Vienna: IAEA).

Irwin, D.J. et al. (1999), *Chemical Incident Management: Public Health Physicians* (London: The Stationery Office).

Jernigan, D.B., Raghunathan, P.L., Bell, B.P., Brechner, R., Bresnitz, E.A., Butler, J.C. et al. and the National Anthrax Epidemiologic Investigation Team (2002), 'Investigation of bioterrorism-related anthrax, United States, 2001: epidemiologic findings'. *Emerging Infectious Diseases* 8: 1019–28.

Kash, T. and Darling, J. (1998), 'Crisis management: prevention, diagnosis and intervention'. *Leadership and Organisation Development Journal* 19(4): 179–86.

Lerbinger, O. (1997), *The Crisis Manager: Facing Risk and Responsibility* (New York: LEA).

Levinson, J. and Granot, H. (2002), *Transportation Disaster Response Handbook* (London: Academic Press).

London Emergency Services Liaison Panel (LESLP) (2003), *Major Incident Procedure Manual* (London: Directorate of Public Affairs, Metropolitan Police Service).

McColl, N.P. and Prosser, S.L. (2002), *Emergency Data Handbook*. NRPB-W19 (Didcot: National Radiological Protection Board).

Ministry of Civil Defence & Emergency Management (MCDEM) (2002), *Working Together: Developing a CDEM Group Plan* (Wellington: MCDEM).

Ministry of Civil Defence & Emergency Management (MCDEM) (2005), *Focus on Recovery: A Holistic Framework for Recovery in New Zealand* (Wellington: MCDEM).

Mitroff, I. and Pearson, C.M. (1993), *A Diagnostic Guide for Improving Your Organisation's Preparedness* (San Francisco: Jossey-Bass).

NHS Executive (1999), *Clinical Governance in the New NHS* (HSC 1999/065, 16 March 1999).

National Audit Office (2002), *Facing the Challenge: NHS Emergency Planning in England* (Report by the Comptroller and Auditor General HC 36 Session 2002–2003: 15 November 2002) (London: The Stationery Office).

Nicols, M. (2003), *Personal Communication.*

Norman, S. (2002), *Coordination of Emergency Management Strategies between First Responders in London and Central Government: A Critical Assessment* (unpublished MSc thesis) (Coventry: Coventry University).

Ogrizek, M. and Guillery, J.-M. (1999), *Communicating in Crisis: A Theoretical and Practical Guide to Crisis Management* (New York: Aldine de Gruyter).

Okumura, T. et al. (1998), 'The Tokyo Subway Sarin Attack: Disaster Management, Part 1: Community Emergency Response'. *Academic Emergency Medicine* 5(6): 613–17.

Payne, C.F. (1994), 'Handling the Press'. *Disaster Prevention and Management: An International Journal* 3(1): 24–32.

Quarantelli, E. (1998), *What is a Disaster?* (London: Routledge).

Rowe, A. (2003), *Personal Correspondence.*

St Bartholomew's and the Royal London Trust (2003), *Hospital Major Incident Plan* (London: St Bartholomew's and the Royal London Trust).

Simpson, J. (2003), *The Health Protection Agency: An Introduction for the Emergency Planning Community* (London: Health Protection Agency).

Smith, D. and Elliott, D. (2000), *Moving Beyond Denial: Exploring the Barriers to Organisational Learning* (Working Paper 1) (Sheffield: Sheffield University Management School, Centre for Risk and Crisis Management).

Torok, T.J., Tauxe, R.V., Wise, R.P., Livengood, J.R., Sokolow, R., Mauvais, J.A. et al. (1997), 'A large community outbreak of salmonellosis caused by intentional contamination of restaurant salad bars'. *Journal of the American Medical Association* 278: 389–95.

Tucker, W.R. (1999), *Disasters and Emergencies: Managing the Response* (Leicester: Institution of Fire Engineers).

Turney, S. (1990), 'The new FCDA powers: constraints and possibilities'. In *Disaster Planning for the 1990s* (London: London Emergency Planning Information Centre), 110–30.

Waspe, S. (2003), 'STEP 123'. *Chemical Incident Report* 28: 28.

Wheatley, S. (2003), *PCT Assessment Tool* (unpublished report) (Birmingham: Health Protection Agency).

Wheeler H. (1999), 'Chemical terrorism: the Japanese experience and lessons learnt.' *Chemical Incident Report* 14: 10–12.

World Health Organisation (1996), *Community Emergency Preparedness Manual* (Geneva: WHO).

World Health Organisation (2002), *Disasters and Emergencies Training Package* (Addis Ababa: Pan African Emergency Training Centre/WHO).

Index

Page numbers in *italic* refer to the definitions found in the Glossary.
The use of **bold** type indicates major treatment of a subject.